The
Compassionate Sleep Solution:

Calming the Cry

sleeping babies...happy parents

By Eileen Henry

Formatting by
Be More of You Media

Visit Eileen online at
compassionatesleepsolutions.com

Contents

Part 1: Learning The Method

By the end of this chapter you will know how to let go – with confidence.

4. Understanding The Cry – *Without Going Insane!*
Understand that crying is often a much bigger problem for the parent than the child.
- Understand the different kinds of crying. All cries sound alike at 3 a.m.
- Learn to objectively listen to the cry and differentiate between struggle and actual distress.

By the end of this chapter you will be able to discern what crying needs attending to and what crying is struggle and will result in sleep.

5. Self-Soothing For Parents – *Ommmmm…*
Understand how to create a serene environment.
- Learn mindfulness exercises.
- Use breathing and centering to create equanimity.

By the end of this chapter you will be able to care for your child in a manner that creates the calmest emotional environment.

6. Make Sex A Priority – *Your relationship depends on it!*
You already know how great sex is; you already understand why it is important for your marriage.
- Understand that you can have a baby and still find time for sex.
- Make a plan for reactivating your sex life.

By the end of this chapter you will make sex an important part of your dependable and predicable routine.

Part 2: Action Plan - 3 Steps To Peaceful Rest

7. Create Your Best Sleep Environment – *Both physical and emotional!*

Understand that there are two sleep environments: *The Physical* and *The Emotional*.

- Create the best physical environment
- Create the most supportive emotional environment

By the end of this chapter you will be able to create the environment most conducive to quality sleep.

8. Create A Routine – *Your baby wants consistency!*

Learn how a consistent routine can turn chaos into calm!

- Show your baby what happens next within a context they can understand
- Show your baby when sleep happens

By the end of this chapter, you will have created a routine that will help your baby prepare for sleep.

9. Begin With A Dress Rehearsal – *Say it, mean it, show it, do it!*

Show your baby the new way of sleep.

- Do a walk through with your child. This is as important for you as it is to your baby.

By the end of this chapter you will know exactly how to introduce your child to the new way of sleep.

Part 3: Finding Success – Opening Night and Follow Through

10. Put It All Together - *Opening Night!*

Put into action everything you have learned in this book.

- Understand that you must remain consistent for this process to work.
- Do sleep this way for the next 3 years.

By the end of this chapter you will understand how to get sleep on track and keep it that way.

11. Ongoing Success: Make Naps A Priority – *Never give up!*

Follow this process every day until you get naps

- Understand that naps are harder and take longer

By the end of this chapter you will understand how to make naps possible.

12. In Conclusion - Nighty Night

You made it! You now have the tools for a great night's sleep...for you and your little one.

Sweet dreams!

The Compassionate Sleep Solution

Dear Parent,

You are not bad or wrong for having ended up on your current path of sleep. Chances are you are here because you have done everything right for your newborn baby.

You are reading this book because you are a good and loving parent. Wanting better and more dependable sleep for yourself and your child is a loving thought. Wanting to make the changes to achieve this is a loving act.

I invite you to drop your guilt here. Guilt will not serve you in this process. It is a natural part of parenting and an unfortunate part of humanness that gets in our way. Focusing on sleep as being a gift to your child and your family is a much more useful mindset for going forward and making healthy changes.

My goal is to reframe some of your thoughts around the problems that you are facing in getting better sleep. Having worked with families on sleep for almost two decades, I am fully aware of what gets in the way of better sleep. I faced the same blocks and hurtles.

I hope that The Compassionate Sleep Solution provides you with a repeatable and sustainable way of doing sleep. This is a process that your baby will come to recognize and believe it or not – appreciate.

Warm regards,
Eileen Henry, Compassionate Sleep Solutions

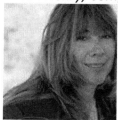

How To Use This Book

Here is your invitation to better and more restful sleep.

If you have gotten this far, chances are your sleep is compromised and you are looking for solutions.

I hope *The Compassionate Sleep Solution* inspires you to look at your child as a competent individual and capable of learning the skills described in these pages. I hope that once you are done, you take your enthusiasm to your child and let him/her see how excited you are to finally get some rest.

Upon finishing this book, I hope you feel confident in what you have learned and practiced as a result. With the tools and practices you learn remember that YOU are enough. Your comforting and loving presence will usher your child through the necessary changes and what you provide will be enough to achieve peaceful and rejuvenating sleep.

Read this book in order. Understanding each aspect of the process is important to the final stage of **Putting it All Together**.

There are four major sleep methods:

Cry It Out (CIO) – a deal breaker for most parents. It works for many and therefore pediatricians recommend it because their best evidence scientific conclusion is that there is no evidence of harm. However, as pointed out to me by one of my clients, *no evidence of harm is different than evidence of NO harm.* Fortunately, we have evolved since the cave and so have our babies. We are not leaving them alone to cry. There is a better way than cry it out. Compassionate Sleep Solutions is that way.

Stay and pay – This is what I call the "listening until you sleep" approach. Many parents insist on staying in the presence and supporting their child through all of their child's upsets, struggles, and cries. I say, "Rock on." This approach works best from 0-4 months of age. In fact, I often recommend this with younger babies since most of us are still co-sleeping (room sharing or bed-sharing) at this age. At 5-8 months, this can increase crying. You aren't doing anything wrong; it is just that your baby is too smart. You are the object of his/her desire and they tend to cry at us until they get what they want. They want us to fix it.

A variation on the CIO: Cry It Out, theme – I've found most parents take this approach. They feel too horrible about saying, "Goodnight, see you in the morning." After going out and suffering from a panic attack listening to the cry, it is understandably hard to face night number two. Therefore, parents feel better doing check-ins. However, the child is unprepared, the parent is unprepared, and it all goes to hell night one and parents return to the sleep crutches (explained in depth throughout this book). This is where we can unintentionally train the child to cry. Because parents go in, the cycle of crying starts over again. If you fall back on the sleep crutches, it significantly increases future crying, making starting over and trying without the crutches that much harder. There is a better way...

The Compassionate Sleep Solution – This is what you're learning in this book! A way to be present and loving, yet allow your child to gain confidence and autonomy. Skills that will help them later in life! Read on...

I would like to invite you to see this as a simple process. There are only a few ideas that you need to embrace to see sleep in a different light.

Chapter 1

Understanding Your Baby's Basic Needs

In this chapter, you will learn:

How to figure out the difference between a want and a need for your baby.

Understanding authentic needs and how to meet those needs.

Knowing your part in what I call "parent-reinforced-needs" and how you may have created a sleepcrutch that your baby no longer needs.

Why it matters:

By eliminating the sleep crutch that is a want and not a need will get everyone a great night's sleep!

Part 1: Learning The Method

1. Understanding Your Baby's Basic Needs

This chapter is to reassure you that there are typically only a handful of true, genuine needs we are providing for during the day. There are true needs, and there are needs that we (parents) create. Each day I hear parents say, *"My baby needs me to hold his hand to sleep or my baby needs me to nurse him to sleep."* The language we use is important in understanding the truth. The truth is that your baby now thinks he needs this, when in fact he wants it. Seeing these authentic needs and parent-created needs as separate will help you understand your part in what your child needs from you in order to learn the developmental skill of sleep. We are not wrong for giving our infants what they want. In fact doing so at birth is in part how we create a secure attachment and bond (the primary and most important need).

The Strength of Being Separate

The fundamental strength in going to sleep is separateness. Your baby needs to learn that it is OK to be apart, that they are safe, loved, and if a real problem occurs, you will be there. As they learn this, they will also come to learn that there is contentment in separateness. It is a happy day when a parent hears their infant cooing happily and drifting off to sleep.

There Are Two Kinds of Needs:

- **Basic** - The basic needs common to all babies.

- **Parent Reinforced** - Needs that you, as a parent, have created early on, when your baby needed your support. But, as your baby develops, they can – and should – outgrow these needs.

What are the Basic Needs?

For our purposes in regulating your child's sleep, we need only focus on four:

- Good Love
- Good Nutrition
- Good Play
- Good Sleep

Our children are learning how to care for themselves, in part, by how we care for them. They will mostly learn by watching us care for ourselves around these basic needs.

They are watching *everything*. Much like the NSA.

Basic Need #1: Love

Love is all you need...

Love and compassion are what you will continue to use to support your child in everything they do - every struggle, every disturbance, every joy - forever and ever, amen. Love includes many values that you want to model for your child. I believe respect is at the top of the list. We respect the self by tending to the following needs in a mindful, intentional, and gentle way. What do you want to show your child in regards to self-care and love?

Love is the most powerful presence in sleep. I do not believe that you must be physically connected to your child (or anyone for that matter!) to assure that love is felt. Remember, "L is for the way you look at me." Here is a simple acronym I like for LOVE:

L – Is for the way you remain **lovingly** connected and responsive to your child during this transition and throughout the night.

O – Is for your **omnipresence**. You will fulfill your child's assumption in that your primary parental purpose on this planet is to respond to and fulfill her every need (children do not know the difference between a want/desire and a need. This is a learned concept. Teach your children well...).

V – Is for the **very extraordinary bond and healthy attachment** that you have worked so hard to establish. Trust that it will not be broken in the learning of this vitally important health skill. When we remain consistent and attentive there is no way we can compromise this strong bond. In fact, this process strengthens the bond.

E – Is for **empathy and emotional attunement**. This supports the unwavering fact that you are even more empathetic and emotionally attuned to your baby than anyone that you adore.

It takes one skill to accomplish autonomous and skilled sleep for children - falling. Sometimes when children fall, they cry. Crying happens. You have a kid and kids cry – accept it.

Crying – Embrace It and Support The Cry

Crying is the number one thing parents are trying to avoid. It makes sense. Now that we are parents, part of our concern is identifying the cause of crying and solving the problem. For most of us that means – stop the damn crying. I'm here to tell you. **"Crying is OK!"** It doesn't feel OK, but it is one of the ways your child has to communicate their needs to you. It doesn't benefit you to relate your child's crying with a lack of love. Being present and attuned to our child in all of their emotional states is an act of love.

The need for a regulated, accurate mirror:

Imagine you are a baby in a crib, you are crying and your caregiver comes into your field of view. What do you see on that person's face? Is it anger, frustration and despair? Or is it calm loving concern? You are your child's mirror and how you react to your baby's cry will help establish a behavioral pattern that will be with them for the rest of their life!

Compassionate Sleep Solutions will offer you the most extensive crying reduction program that you will find. No Cry sleep solutions are great - in theory.

- My goal is to prepare you for reality.
- My goal is to prepare you and your child in a way that will significantly reduce the crying.
- Your responsiveness and consistent connection to your child as he learns this new skill will further reduce your child's crying.

However, this is the truth: Crying happens, and it happens because crying is a healthy response to loss. As it relates to sleep, our child is experiencing the loss of the sleep crutch. He doesn't know how to do this any other way. He thinks he needs that crutch. To "fall" without the crutch feels strange, unfamiliar, and foreign. He is tired and frustrated. This is hard. I do not believe he is scared. He knows where he is and he knows he is safe and loved. The person who is scared is you and it's OK that you are scared.

Basic Need #2: Nutrition

If you are starting to make changes in infancy, meeting your baby's nutritional needs in the night is part of sleep. I will discuss feedings in the night under each stage of development. For now, think of your baby's age and weight, then consider what his authentic need for food might be throughout the night. Most of us know when we are being used as a pacifier.

Hint: If he is over 8 months old, healthy, and devouring solid food during the day, chances are you can pass the focal feed section and go directly to night weaning. The feeding relationship is a personal one. However, you can attend to this need AND get quality sleep.

Basic Need #3: Play

The first decade of the child's life is devoted solely to play. They are learning everything through their experiences, their daily associations and play. It is almost like a full-time job. Offering plenty of opportunity in the routine of the day for uninterrupted, child-directed, child-initiated and open-ended play is a great way to meet this need in your child. By incorporating this type of play into your daily routine, at naptime or at the end of the day when your child has had the other basic needs satisfied, even young babies will recognize this same type of autonomy and come to find contentment in this quality time.

Basic Need #4: Sleep

Sleep begets sleep. This is one thing that all sleep specialists agree on. The better quality and quantity of day sleep your baby gets, the better his night sleep will be. This is what this book is about.

What do you want to teach your child about the value of sleep?

What is a Parent-Reinforced Need?

Understanding the parent-reinforced need – An important part of the process of developing better sleep habits is understanding the role you have played in either creating a need or reinforcing a need that your baby has outgrown. In other words, you have created a cause and effect feedback loop.

This is how a feedback loop is created:

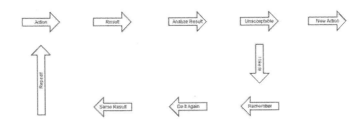

1. The child has an impulse/desire/request – they cry.
2. We meet that with a response – we show up and we do something or offer something say, rocking or feeding.
3. Each time we hear the cry - we rock...
4. As we repeat our response, we create an expectation.
5. Crying = rocking. Your baby thinks, "If I cry – they rock."
6. As we repeat our response to the expectation, the expectation becomes a need.
7. The child comes to believe that they need to be rocked in order to go to sleep.

Understand that you have created the need based on your actions. Your child is sleep training you! This book will retrain you. We are not bad or wrong for doing what we have done. We only need to have the awareness of what we did. What choices and actions did we make that contributed to where we are now? It is only from this awareness that we can begin to undo what was done. Undoing = new choices.

We are mommies and daddies, dammit. We are going to fix things. However, the more we do for them, the less they can do for themselves. If we want to change anything we are doing with our children, we do need to show them in a consistent and understandable way what the new paradigm will be.

Parent Reinforced Need #1: Crutches

A crutch is a something we use to help carry our baby over the bridge to sleep. Crutches are good and useful tools at first. When needed, crutches keep us from falling. However, a time will come when we need to set them aside so that our children can learn the developmental skill of falling as applied to the sleep process. Here is a list of what we do to "fix" the "falling" of "falling asleep":

- Nurse
- Hold
- Bounce
- Rock
- Walk
- Pacifier
- Swing
- Sway
- Shush
- Drive
- Stroll
- Swaddle
- Pat
- Touch

When we fix the falling with any of the crutches listed above, we reinforce the need for the child to have these conditions in order to get to sleep.

Therefore, when your baby comes to light sleep or has natural wakeful periods in the night, you will need to provide this condition in order for your child to return to sleep. This can be many times in the night, often lasting all night long. Exhaustion on the part of new parents can lead to anxiety, depression, and the thinking of *bad thoughts*. And this isn't going to be good for anyone.

Parent Reinforced Need #2: Associations

Your child is learning everything through association.

You can continue to use the main association that your child has learned to relate to sleep. And that is YOU!

- Your presence
- Your touch
- Your voice
- Your face
- Your love

Parent Reinforced Need #3: Your love is enough!

Our job as parents is to accompany our child to the footbridge of sleep. Their job is to cross over.

We hold their hands and bring them to the bridge in these ways:

- Creating a recognizable routine of the day around sleep and the other basic needs;

- Preparing them at night with proper quality time with us;
- Providing a lovely ritual that is calming and readies the brain for sleep;
- Placing them at the foot of the bridge into the sleep place and allowing them to cross over.

During sleep they will come back halfway across the bridge as they travel in and out of light sleep cycles. When sleep is handled in this manner, we do not have to drag our butts off our own bridge to come and carry them back over theirs all night long.

You can continue to feed your baby...just not all the way to sleep. You can continue to hold your baby...just not all the way to sleep. You can continue to be present with your baby...just not until she is all the way and over the bridge and asleep.

Why Understanding The Needs Are Important to Sleep

Understanding your baby's basic needs and how they influence sleep will help you in getting more sleep. It will keep you focused on what is important and make this process simple, doable, and repeatable.

People come to me when they have enmeshed the three parent reinforced needs listed above in the previous section.

- Love/relationship – holding to sleep, rocking to sleep, in physical contact with infant in order to sleep.
- Food/nutrition – feeding to sleep.

This is natural and normal for newborn babies (0-4 months). The enmeshment or entanglement of the eat, love, sleep relationship is the no-fail set up for establishing the healthy bond.

However, after this newborn stage, you will want to consider unraveling this enmeshment. This book will help you in unraveling and untangling the enmeshment of the basic needs. These can facilitate sleep at first. However, if we use them for longer than developmentally necessary, they can interrupt sleep and the sleep process. Here's how:

- It takes longer and longer to put your baby all the way to sleep.
- It quits working all together. You finally get the child to sleep and as soon as her back hits the bed her eyes fly open and she looks at you as if to say, "Seriously? You *are* kidding, right?"
- You are terrified of the inevitable dead-end but you don't know what to do. Therefore, you continue repeating the same actions over and over, hoping for a different outcome. This is the classic definition of insanity.

Here is what your baby can learn:

- Food, relationship and play are for the waking hours.
- Only sleep is happening during sleep time.

Using any method necessary to "put our child to sleep" is what I refer to as sleep crutches.
They are also commonly referred to as props, conditions and sleep associations.

If you want to you can.

I am just here to tell you that you don't have to.

It is fine to fix newborn sleep.
It is fine to allow our babies to learn a new way to sleep that does not involve our fixing.
They can all learn to fall asleep on their own...with our help.

And it is fine until THREE things happen:

- You either can't fix it;
- You don't want to fix it anymore or;
- Your child is capable of more.

Fixing his sleep and allowing him to fall all over the place in all of these other venues is fine.
Fixing all of it is not.

A parent does not have to hold the fantasy that their child will be able to perform many tasks. We hold our children for months and never doubt the fact that they will stand up and walk away from us. In doing so, they will have to fall and get up again many, many times. However, the idea that they will be able to fall asleep seems impossible.

Babies four to six months old are capable of learning when, where and how their basic needs are attended to each day. Please pay close attention to the Routine section of this book for more instruction on this.

What Your Baby is Capable of at Each Stage of Development:

While considering the needs of your baby, here is what they should be capable of as infant and toddlers. Your mileage may vary, so don't worry if your child is a little ahead or behind this schedule.

Newborn: 0-5 months
- Your newborn is learning the difference between night and day.
- You are focusing on bonding with your baby.
- Your baby can sleep any time anywhere.
- Your baby may sleep a lot during the day.
- Your baby may sleep very little one day and a lot the next.
- Your baby may look like he doesn't sleep much at all.
- Your baby needs more soothing and help sleeping than he will ever need again in his life.
- Your newborn has a need for frequent naps during the day.
- Your newborn has a need for frequent feedings in the day and night.
- Sleep is all over the place.
- At 3-5 months your newborn is transitioning into the first stage of infancy.
- At 3-5 months your baby is able to learn the skill of falling asleep.
- Between 5-6 months of age your baby's self-soothing mechanism is stable. Please refer to my blog post <u>They Are Stronger Than We Think</u> for more information.

Easy as pie right?

Infancy: 5 – 10 months

- Your infant can learn the skill of falling asleep and returning to sleep at this stage.

- Most 5 to 7 month old babies need only one feeding in the night.
- Once your baby starts a regular daily diet of solid food, the overriding need at night is to rest the digestive system.
- Night weaning based on the infant's food need can happen easily between 8 - 10 months.

Toddlers – 10 months to 3 years

- By this stage your infant is falling in his waking world.
- How we respond or react to daytime falling, as you know, makes a difference to their own reactions to their falls.
- Our reaction to night falling has a similar affect. A calm response is our goal.
- Therefore, falling asleep and sleeping through the night is a reality all toddlers can accomplish.
- Parents still might need to respond occasionally to night awakenings and offer supportive check-ins.
- Your child has made a major cognitive leap by this stage. She now understands probability of outcome based on cause and effect.
- She knows her cry causes an effect in you.
- You can remain responsive to her cries and emotionally connected without fixing sleep.

Chapter 2

Understand Your Baby's Development – *Will she ever sleep through the night?*

In this chapter, you will learn:

• How the development of the child is the most interruptive to sleep during the first three years.
• Sleep regressions are developmental leaps.
• Transforming challenges into advantages at each stage of development.

Why it matters:

By the end of this chapter you will understand that whatever happens in the crib is normal and you don't have to rescue them from every little thing.

2. Understand Your Baby's Development – *"Will she ever sleep through the night?"*

Stages Of Development:

No matter how you have handled sleep, no matter what success you have experienced, no matter where you are in the process – development will come along and change it all. The underlying development that accompanies teething, travel, illness and life's twists and turns is the single most interruptive thing to sleep. The good news is that you can get back on track; the better news is sleep will return, the bad news is that it is up to you to make it happen. The good and bad news is that this is not magic.

Child development is the physical, biological, psychological and emotional changes that occur in human beings between birth and the end of adolescence, as the individual progresses from dependency to increasing autonomy. It is a continuous process with a predictable sequence yet having a unique course for every child.

The important takeaway is "continuous process" and "increasing autonomy." Development is ongoing and never-ending. However, development in the first three years is explosive (not to mention expulsive). Your baby is busy!

- Your baby was born with only 25% of his adult brain mass.
- Even though infancy is only 2% of our lifespan, 80% of your baby's total brain growth will happen by the time she is two.
- In the first year alone, your baby will increase from 25% to 60% volume of the adult brain.

19

- That is almost 2/3 total growth of the brain occurring in this very short window.
- When your child turns three he will have grown 90% of his adult brain.

Getting enough sleep during this rapid growth period is essential. This can be frustrating for new parents, as they find themselves on the giving end of the spectrum (for *years*), while getting nothing back. Kind of like in-laws (outlaws, at least, are *wanted*). Focusing on the following list in the first few years of development can simplify your life. Much has been written about the "overscheduled child." It is not good and will get in the way of sleep. This will leave you with a short list of questions. Your answers could provide your child the optimum conditions for excellent brain development.

So what feeds this rapidly growing brain?

Sleep
- Is my child getting enough sleep?
- Is it high quality sleep or interrupted sleep? (They can handle more interruptions than we can).

Experience
- Am I being mindful of the experiences I offer my child? Is it enough? Is it too much? (The growing brain can be over stimulated easily and that can affect both day and night sleep in the early years.)

Nutrition
- What do I want to teach my child in regards to nutrition?
- Am I feeding them based on an authentic need for food or for comfort?

Love
- Does my child need to be physically connected to my body 24/7 in order to feel my love?

All of the above can have an impact on sleep. This is why I am a pusher of peace and the concept of less being more. Slow down, do less and let the child fully experience their natural environment. Less stuff, less activity, less running about is my bias for the early months/years. Of course, keep in mind the predilections of the individual child. I often have very active parents who wonder how they are going to fit a small child into their activities. Pay attention to your child and see. Your child will tell you if it is too much. Some children need more; some children need less. Trust yourself to know where your child falls on that continuum. Yes, you can likely teach your child to come up to your pace but here is an overriding question that can be applied to so much:

Just because we *can* do something, does it mean we *should*?

Why Is Development Important?

Your child's growth, coupled with learning the basic skill set that will carry your child through life, is the most interruptive to sleep.

- **Development is the single most disruptive force on child sleep.**
- **Development is most disruptive during the first three years.**
- **Sleep is a developmental skill.**
- **All development affects sleep in both positive and challenging ways.**

Your child is now learning skills (gross motor, fine motor, language, etc.) for the first time which will carry her through life. In this learning, the brain is very busy. Brain activity goes on all night long as new information and learning passes through the networks and pathways of the brain, becoming imprinted into memory. The human brain is a *learning machine.* Up until around the age of 5, it literally *rewires* itself in response to new information. It can help parents to know that much of what is going on in the crib is normal and healthy, and our job can simply be to step back and let it happen. Remember that everything your child is learning during the day your child is also practicing in the night.

We celebrate the developmental milestones in our child's life, yet these milestones can be very disruptive to sleep. This is OK!

How Does Development Affect Your Child's Sleep?

Here is a list of developmental milestones that can disrupt sleep:

- Transition out of swaddle
- Going from back to belly and getting stuck there
- Going from back to belly and then back to back again
- Rolling
- Crawling
- Sitting
- Standing
- Cruising
- Walking
- Fine motor skills and the ability to remove clothing or perhaps a diaper and soil the sheets.
- Climbing
- Talking
- Growth spurts
- Teething

Parents often put growth spurts and teething at the top of the list. I intentionally put them at the bottom of the list. Growth spurts and teething happen in conjunction with other development. I find the underlying development much more interruptive. When a child knows how to negotiate the "falling" of falling asleep, I often find that growth spurts and teething are not as disruptive as we might think.

Sometimes we get what I call the **Perfect Storm of Sleep Interruptions**.
A huge developmental shift + teething + travel + illness + any big change in the child's world = **HUGE** sleep disruption.

Understanding that development in and of itself is the number one cause of sleep disruptions will help you in navigating these times with consistency and responsiveness.

Why is understanding development important to sleep?

- This understanding will help you make changes at any age and under any developmental occurrence.
- This understanding will help you maintain the changes as your child grows.
- This understanding will help you remain consistent yet flexible as the new skills your child is practicing in the waking hours show up in the crib at night.
- This understanding will help you realize that **almost** everything in regards to sudden changes and or "regressions" are a normal part of this development.

If I could really get parents to understand how the explosion of brain development and child development impacts sleep, then NOTHING they witness would surprise them. I do not know why, but in regards to child sleep this is one of the most difficult concepts for parents to fully understand. Even with this knowledge, development coupled with the natural and ongoing disruptions of sleep is the most difficult concept to fully accept.

But I will tell you this; development, thank goodness, is not dependent on either our understanding or accepting it. It is an ongoing, unstoppable process. It is like standing on the beach and trying to keep the waves from rolling in or the tide from going out.

Development, although ongoing and progressive, is not linear. It looks like this:

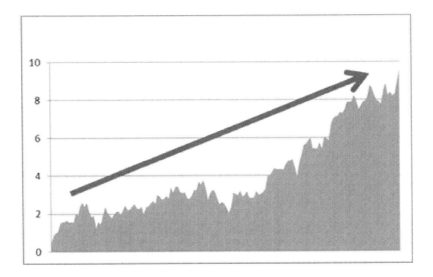

On and on...over and over...for decades to come.

Sleep is a learned skill

I do not call what we do "sleep training." We do not have to train a human how to sleep. We do have to offer them the opportunities and the environment to be able to sleep. We do have to offer them the opportunity and the environment to learn the skill of sleep. We do this by not fixing the falling with the sleep crutches I have already mentioned. This is how we move toward mastering any skill

1. First we learn the skill – This takes a certain amount of frustration and struggle.
2. Secondly we repeat this newly learned skill – Practice is the only way to master anything.
3. Lastly we master any skill by the continued repetition

Sleep like all development looks exactly like the chart above in the first few years as well because learning to sleep is a developmental process that happens over time. Your baby's sleep is affected by all other development in this period of massive and rapid brain growth.

Regression Is a Necessary and Important Part Of Development

Although the way regression shows up in the bed/crib around sleep is disappointing, it is part of the development in sleep as well as all other development. During development and learning a new skill, the brain is in a constant back and forth between equilibrium and disequilibrium, balance and imbalance, synchrony and asynchrony, regulation and dis-regulation.

During development and learning a new skill the brain will go back to what it already knows. The brain seeks to do what it already knows how to do with ease in order to leap ahead into the new territory of the unknown. We notice this when toddlers start to walk. They will go back and only crawl for a week or more. It is important for the brain and body to do this. It is important for us to let them do this.

This "going back" can look like a regression and is often talked about as the sleep regressions that happen at fairly predictable times as the brain wakes up:

- 3 month

- 6 month
- 9 month

I encourage you to look at these and rejoice. Generally, right after a regression they do something amazing and new...like pull an 8 hour stretch of sleep. Or get up and walk across the house and clean the kitchen after dinner. Well, at some point they will. One can dream.

What to do about development?

Once the interruption of development is understood, what can a parent do to get enough sleep in spite of it?

- Keep reading and increase your understanding of development.
- Trust that development is a healthy part of growing and adopt the "this too shall pass" mentality.
- Get out of the way and let it happen.
- Do not take your child's development personally. In other words, get over yourself.
- Are you a fan of roller coasters? Expect anything and everything and stay on course. See graph above. This ride is a lot easier said than done.
- Hold a loving and safe space for development to happen in.
- In educational terms it is called scaffolding. We support the building blocks of development without holding up the whole building.
- Hone your acceptance skills.
- Hone your sensitive observation skills.
- Hone your self-regulation skills. In other words, try not to unravel so.
- Do what is outlined in this book in the order that it is presented.

- Do it over and over again no matter what.
- Feel free to go in and offer reassurance.

What to expect when they/we are developing.

We are developing along with our child. The later stages of autonomy, interdependence, individuation, and differentiation take a lifetime. Regressions are ongoing in the parent as well as the child. Check the toddler section below and then do a self-check. We too will regress. Becoming self-aware is the only way to progress. This is progress not perfection.

We are continually being mindful of the child's perspective while trying NOT to sink to their developmental level. But we are not perfect. At some point our inner toddler shows up. So be it. Acknowledge her, empathize with her and reassure her.
Then put her (your) ass to bed.

What to expect at the following stages of development:

0-4 months – The Newborn
- Sleep is literally all over the place both physically and timing wise.
- Naps are short or long - both are normal.
- They can sleep constantly or hardly at all - both are typical.
- Notice the time between sleep periods (see napping chart). Newborns can handle about an hour awake before they are ready to sleep again.
- When they are coming up to 3-4 months, get the location consistent. In other words, "Do sleep in the sleep place."
- Co-sleeping is great and close proximity makes life easy.
- This is when unintentional bed-sharing is most likely to happen.

- Feedings are frequent and there are a lot of night wakings or they pull an 8-hour stretch.
- The important thing is that everything will change so don't let it freak you out.
- This is the time where an incremental approach is the most possible.
- This can be a good time to allow your baby to start learning the falling of falling asleep.
- 3-4 months is the first brain wake up and your baby becomes more interactive. They smile, giggle, coo and start what is a back and forth repeating of these sounds. Their focus is further out and they quite literally look more awake.
- This brain wake up can happen in the night and quite suddenly, as in overnight, your baby starts waking every hour again.

5-7 months – The Infant

- Naps consolidate into 3 per day (see napping chart for timings in between naps)
- The brain wake-up at this stage can be profound. A wakeful brain means your baby can start waking every hour at night again.
- This is the best time to allow your baby to learn to fall asleep.
- This is a great time to transition your baby out of the family bed and into a bassinet or into her own room.
- Once your baby is falling sleep on her own with you out of the room, start working on lengthening naps.
- It is best if naps look, feel, smell, and sound just like night sleep
- This is when parents notice that going in to offer support can increase crying. This is normal. Your baby is smarter now and

more aware. Hold on to yourself and remain present and centered.

- Offer love and support without fixing or rescuing.

8-10 months – Last Stage of Infancy

- Naps consolidate into two naps a day (see chart for timings and time awake between naps)
- The third brain wake up. Welcome to 35% of adult brain mass. You are in the presence of a new and growing brilliance.
- Your baby understands probability of outcome based on cause and effect with the accuracy of a scientist.
- This is when your data needs to become rock solid. *I come. I go. I offer support. I do not fix your sleep or rescue you out of sleep because you know what to do in that crib and you know how to be content in that space.*
- If you do the focal feed and feed your baby based on authentic need for hunger rather than "mommy as human pacifier," this is when infant led night weaning is most likely to happen. (The Focal Feed is discussed at length in Chapter 3)
- If you were a human pacifier, this is when most babies do not need feeding in the night.
- This is when **you** can do night weaning. This is when you can release the barnacle from the mothership.
- This is when your baby's solid food intake increases and does not slow down until they are in their 20's (or 240 months of age.)
- This stage is often talked about as the "hands off, don't even try sleep training due to the dreaded 9-month regression" phase of development. I don't agree with this philosophy.
- Do not be afraid. This is when your baby will understand the preparation part of the sleep plan even more.

- This is when your baby is learning some language and understands you. After all, you have been talking to your baby from birth.
- This is when your baby is moving away from you (crawling) and your communication system is in place so you can warn him if he is headed for a cliff.
- This is when your baby understands separateness because he is moving in and out of it all day long
- This is when your baby understands that your coming and going is not abandonment, neglect, or trauma because for 8-10 solid months you have not abandoned, neglected or traumatized him once. Ever. (Crying is not trauma - it's a natural part of expression. Watch *The Notebook* for more information about crying.)
- This is when your baby can do the falling of falling asleep 100% of the time, by herself, in her sleep place, with your loving support, coming and going from a place in the house. Your baby understands physical environment and the emotional context of that environment.
- This is when your baby drops the third nap
- This is when bedtime moves up to a much earlier time because, given the list above, your baby is exhausted.
- This is when sleeping through the night becomes a beautiful reality ☺

11 months – 3.5 years – The Toddler

- This is when your baby becomes upright and starts to walk and run about this earth
- This is another major brain wake-up. Your baby's brain is lit up like a Christmas tree.
- This is when they transition to one nap (15 months to 2 years)

- This transition can take a month. Once again, move up bedtime a bit earlier.
- This is where they can flat out resist naps altogether.
- This is when the will of the child rises. This is hard. This is challenging. We remain consistent, loving, and hold the boundaries.
- This is the new and improved cry. It looks like screaming yelling kicking screaming banging throwing and it can trigger a deep desire in the adult to do the same.
- This brain state is the chemical state of falling in love. Remember that? When you had little to no appetite (for food) and you felt great on 3 hours of sleep?
- This is when sleep seemingly goes to hell in a toy basket.
- Your baby is falling in love with you. She is developing interpersonal communication, play habits, and the pursuit of new and enriching experiences.
- This is when your baby will grow another 45% of brain mass.
- This is when I want you to seriously consider the sensory and emotional experiences you are feeding that growing brain. They might not remember this time but their brain and bodies will. What do we want the subconscious and the unconscious to remember?
- This is when emotions run high. Testing boundaries and loving limits becomes higher and the sleep disruptions are highest.
- This is when you need Janet Lansbury's book *Discipline Without Shame*.
- This is when we show our children lovingly what TO do instead of continually telling them what NOT to do.
- This is when the drive for autonomy is high.
- This is when the icky human feeling of ambivalence creeps in and creates emotional struggle and separation anxiety. "*Should I stay or should I go...should I run away from the*

secure base or climb back up inside of her uterus where the world didn't test me and I didn't feel compelled to test it?"

- This is when your child can handle many problems and is actively seeking them out as a form of learning and expansion. It is at the same time both hilarious and horrifying.
- This is the age where your toddler is going from beginning toddler to accomplished toddler.
- Accomplished toddlers, age 2-4, become skillful at language and therefore become skillful at negotiating, prolonging, insisting and persisting.
- This is when NO becomes a complete sentence.
- This is when toddlers become hijackers and hijack the nighttime ritual. If you have twins this is when you have your own terrorist cell. We do not negotiate with terrorists.
- This is when you begin the long and lifetime practice of not taking your child's brain personally.
- They are not doing this to drive you nuts they are doing this because they can - plain and simple.
- This can be difficult for parents. It feels out of control and adults don't dig that.
- This is how the toddler learns; through repetition. They are running tests on their world. Physical tests, emotional tests and mental tests. It can make us feel mental. If there is a crazy person in the room, make sure it is NOT you. They need us to remain strong and loving.
- They are curious, enthusiastic and smart.
- Their feelings run big and large and they do not have the ability to contain and manage those feelings.
- It is our job to teach them to ride the waves of these feelings.
- It is unsettling and we become afraid. Because we are at the developmental stage of emotions and thoughts. Emotions have a story attached. The story has a foot in the past and a foot in the future. Emotions can take a dump on the now.

- Your toddler is sensation and feelings based. They don't have a story about these feelings. This is in part why they are so happy.
- This is when we have a profound moment to hold the space for them. We are the container.
- The container is neutral, respectful, loving, and supportive.
- The container does not need to make something happen or keep something from happening the container just holds. To do this we **must** hold onto the self.
- This is a beautiful opportunity to impart on your child that feelings are meant to be felt. All feelings are meant to be felt. Simple, not easy I know.
- This is where we confront our own fear, resistance, persistence, and revulsion of negative and uncomfortable emotions.
- This will prepare you for adolescence and I highly suggest that you use this time to prepare. Bigger and bolder is right around the developmental corner.
- This is where we get to be human. We get to mess up. This is when we are most likely to yell at our wide eyed little love.
- This is where we feel the horrible feelings of guilt and remorse. We start a savings plan for therapy. OURS! Because it is not about them it is about us.
- We get to clean up the mess and show our child what repair and clean up looks like.
- Some of the best moments and creations of this lifetime will come right out of a mess.
- Messiness is unavoidable if we are going to live this life to the fullest.

Chapter 3
Prepare to "Let Go" -
The Art of Falling!

In this chapter, you will learn:

Letting go and independently falling asleep is something every baby can learn.

• Believe in your baby. Your baby knows how to sleep.

• All babies are born sleepers, your job is to simply allow your baby to fall.

Why it matters:

Falling is a natural part of development.

Learning how to fall and get up again is one of the best preparations for life.

3. Preparing to "Let Go" - *The Art of Falling*

Learning how to fall is one of the best lessons of life.
                                                        -Magda Gerber

The Art of Falling

We can all fall. We fall asleep, we fall learning to walk, we fall emotionally, we fall in and out of love - *we fall*. Most falling involves uncertainty, uneasiness, new sensations, trust, struggle, and quite often, tears. We will not be there to catch our children every step of the way but we can offer our love and support. The falling of falling to sleep, and being separate is not harmful, traumatic or scary. It is new and unfamiliar. Once learned, it is delightful and lovely. See falling and being separate with new eyes.

The fundamental skill in going to sleep is the art of falling. Falling is that point where we all let go and allow ourselves to cross the bridge from wakefulness to sleep. Adults feel it and we know that sleep is coming. Infants feel it and it stimulates the Moro, or startle reflex. When we nurse our infants to sleep, rock them, hold them, and swaddle them, we fix that falling. It is a kind thing to do for a baby who does not yet have that reflex integrated into his nervous system. However, as they develop and the reflexes integrate, they can learn how to fall. This is the first skill they must learn to become successful autonomous sleepers.

What is falling?

Being able to fall and get up again is a great metaphor for living life to the fullest.

Sleep is a vitally important basic need. Learning to fall asleep and return to sleep is a developmental skill that all children can accomplish:

- Falling asleep is a physical sensation in the body.
- It activates the Moro reflex (startle reflex).
- This reflex is either just beginning to integrate into the nervous system or is newly integrated. (Between 3-6 months)
- This sensation is unfamiliar to the child.

We have all felt it as we drift off to sleep. As we drift into slumber, the body has one final twitch before it relaxes into sleep. Adults understand sleep is coming and relax into the falling because we are familiar with that sensation. We relax, let go, and let sleep. Or if we have had problems with sleep, we get anxious uptight and fight the falling.

This is a new sensation for your baby. This physical sensation of falling is what infants need to experience and master to become skilled sleepers.

It is a sensation that she can and will learn.
- It is a sensation infants can learn at any stage of development.
- "Falling asleep" becomes easier once this reflexive movement has integrated into their nervous system.
- The Moro reflex or startle reflex integrates into the system by 4 - 5 months.

- However, many infants can still negotiate this sensation and "fall asleep" early on (birth - 5 months).

In newborn babies this sensation sometimes stimulates the Moro reflex or startle response. It is kind to help our newborns in the early months fall asleep and part of helping them is to calm down this startle response. Many parents do this by holding, swaddling, rocking, and/or nursing their child to sleep (more on this later).

Falling is a normal part of development.

I invite parents to look at the falling of falling asleep just like any other falling that your child will do as they develop and grow. Here is a list of all the opportunities that your child will have to physically fall in learning a new skill:

- Crawling
- Standing
- Cruising
- Sitting
- Walking
- Running
- Bike riding
- Climbing
- Playing

As your child grows he will have more than ample opportunity to fall:

- Physically
- Mentally
- Emotionally

Why is falling important?

Being able to negotiate this sensation of falling and experience that moment as a relaxing part of the process is very important to sleep. To welcome this surrendering over to the winning side of restful and restorative sleep is what makes us long for bedtime at the end of an exhausting day.

How we as parents adversely impact falling

We fix the falling by doing all of the following until the child is asleep in our arms. Then we put them down to sleep once they are already asleep. If they wake we need to start all over again to fix the falling for them. They simply do not know how to fall because we fix it by doing the following:

- Rock
- Swaddle
- Nurse
- Walk
- Stroll
- Swing
- Bounce
- Drive

We rescue them from falling.

They wake up in the middle of the night and we go and rescue them out of sleep:

- We take them out of the crib and bring them into bed.
- We rock them, nurse them, pat them, bounce them back to sleep when they wake in the night.

- We project emotions onto them such as fear, panic, and trauma (all words I hear each day), and then naturally go to fix it. I hear the craziest nonsense come out of parents' mouths that are all projection.

Why we do it?

We do it mostly because it works. My 13-year old daughter looked at me the other day and said, *"There you go again, Mom. You take a good idea and you run it into the ground."* She is right. If it works I will do it over and over. I am like most of us. I do not change until I have to. Makes sense, no?

We fix child sleep because we learn that this is the way to help infants sleep. We keep doing it because if we don't then the infant looks at us like we are nuts and starts to cry. We fear change and that is human. Even if we are in hell and something clearly needs changing, we are afraid to leave the devil we know for the devil we don't. We also have the tendency to think that when we are in hell we will always be in hell and when we are in heaven we will always be in heaven. Neither is true.

A parent does not have to hold the fantasy that their child will accomplish many complicated tasks. We hold our children for months and never doubt the fact that they will stand up and walk away from us. And in doing so, they will have to fall and get up again many, many times. However, the idea that they will be able to fall asleep seems impossible.

At some point, perhaps sooner than you think, all babies can learn to fall.

At some point we can stop fixing it: What is the truth about the fix?

The more we fix it...
- The more the child comes to expect that we will fix it.
- The more we meet that expectation with the fix.
- The more the child will rely on us to fix their falling.
- The more they rely on it the more we do it.
- The more we do it and the more it works.
- The longer it works the longer we will go without changing things.

I said we fix it. I didn't say we are wrong for fixing it. We fix it because it works. That is smart and adaptive.

However, I am sad to report the fix, as all fixes eventually prove to us, has an inevitable dead end. Quite often when we hit that dead end, the fix is perceived by our little dependent one, as a need.

It is fine to fix newborn sleep.
It is fine to allow our babies to learn a new way to sleep that does not involve our fixing.
They can all learn to fall asleep on their own...with our help.

And fixing is fine until THREE things happen:

1. You can't fix it anymore.
2. You don't want to fix it anymore.
3. Your child is capable of more.

The rest of this book is about un-falling.
Falling do – Do let them fall. If the falling is not dangerous let them fall.
Falling don't – Don't fix all the falling. The more they fall the better they get at falling.

These are techniques that parents can use to facilitate our children in learning how to fall asleep:

- The repetitive movement of putting our infants down increases the familiarity with this sensation.
- Allowing plenty of unrestricted movement free from swaddle.
- Allowing plenty of unrestricted movement free from restraining devices (jumpy seat, exersaucers, carriers, etc.).
- Allowing plenty of floor time where your child is free to move, roll, crawl and experience gross motor development on a hard surface from the position of their backs being flat on the floor.
- As your infant is learning this sensation of falling on the flat surface of the crib placing your hand on the chest with a light pressure can help calm them and ease them into negotiating this falling.
- Do not use crib positioners that force an infant to remain on their back. Once infants can freely move from back to belly to back again let them move in this way. This will help them resettle into sleep.

Good sleepers are made, not born. However, sleep is particularly hard in the following babies.

- Reflux babies.
- Premature babies.
- Babies who have special circumstances at birth - be it health circumstances, trauma or any other issue that either landed your baby in NICU, or experienced other interventions that caused stress for you and/or your baby. Face it. If your baby was stressed, then you were stressed.

If YOU were stressed, then so was your baby.

If your baby falls in to this category you may want to co-sleep for longer and wait to make big changes around sleep. Longer, meaning 6 - 9 months but probably not 1 - 2 years. It depends on how severe the issue is and how much extra soothing your child needs as a result of it.

The Focal Feed

The focal feed was not my brilliant idea. The concept of a "focal feed" came out of research based on newborn infants who were offered a feeding between 10 p.m. and midnight in an effort to increase the length of time they slept without needing to be fed. For all other wake ups, the parents offered what I call "alternate soothing methods." Alternate soothing methods are anything we do to help soothe the infant such as, patting, rocking, and swaying. However, these soothing methods were used to soothe and not to "put" the child all the way into sleep.

Instead of feeding every time the infant woke outside of the 10 p.m. to midnight focal feed time, the parent re-swaddled, held, rocked, and walked the infant instead of feeding.

As a general rule, focal feeds should be done as follows. Times not exact but make note of the range of time you do the focal feedings:

- **0 – 2 Months** - Feed every 1 to 2 hours. Remember, you are creating a bond. You can't love them too much, you can't feed them too much, you can't hold them too much. Respond, respond, respond - that's how you create the bond!
- **3 – 5 Months** - Feedings consolidate into 2 main focal feeds, typically around 11:00 p.m. and after 3:00 a.m.

- **6 – 7 Months** - One feeding after midnight. By this time your baby should be doing 100% of falling asleep by themselves with the exception of the focal feed. If they can go from sleepy to asleep by themselves, they may wake up in the night and if they aren't hungry, they go back to sleep.
- **8 Months -** By 8 months, your child should be able to sleep through the night. In fact, to create a focal feed at this age is almost impossible. Most people get stuck with a 5:00 a.m. feeding. Don't! If you create this habit, it will be extremely difficult to break - leaving for college usually does the trick! Very few mothers heed this warning. Even I did not heed my own warning in this regard. Why would we stop something that works? Why would we not choose the 30-second fix over the 30-minute complaining at 5:00 a.m.? I'll tell you why. If you wait until 9 or 10 months, dropping this feeding can take over a month.

These time frames are typical for most babies, but some children are ahead and some are developmentally behind. For example, a very large baby will have higher caloric needs. There is a movement to begin night weaning your baby and get them sleeping through the night from birth. This is crazy pants! Don't do it.

In my experience as both a mother and as a sleep consultant I have found the following to be true:

- The focal feed works. As shown in the research, most infants are able to go a fairly predictable amount of time without a feeding in the night at certain ages.
- The infant is able to do longer stretches of sleep in the night when they are fed for their authentic need for hunger in the night rather than offering the breast as a pacifier to fix their sleep,

- Infants who are fed based on their authentic need for food have a greater tendency to sleep through or bridge sleep cycles when they are no longer hungry.
- Infants who are offered this "focal feed" tend to self-wean in the night at an earlier stage (some as early as 6-7 months - most between 7-9 months of age).
- The only way to know if they are hungry or are just using the breast as a pacifier is to allow them to fall asleep at the onset of the night AFTER a hearty feed. Then we know they are not hungry and we can allow them to fall asleep without any sleep crutches.
- When the infant learns to fall, they can more easily re-fall (bridge a light sleep cycle or full wake-up) throughout the night.
- This focal feed is more easily established from 0-6 months of age.
- From approximately 8 months on, it is almost impossible to establish a focal feed. Because by this time most infants no longer need to eat in the night.
- By 8 months, I mainly recommend night weaning to reduce the crying in the night.

Establishing a Focal Feed

The ages below offer a guide to the approximate amounts of time a baby can go between feedings in the night. Most mothers have a sense as to when their baby is having a hearty feed and when they are being used as a pacifier.

The only way to allow babies to establish this focal feed is to allow them to "fall asleep" without a sleep crutch at the onset of the night. Once they can fall, babies will return to sleep on their own if they are not truly hungry. As hunger lessens in the night, they are more able to fall back asleep and sleep through the feedings when they are no longer hungry.

- **0-4 months of age** – you can do what I call topping off if your child wakes before you go to bed. However, this is sometimes referred to as a dream feed. I am not a fan of that. It is a dead end. By the time it stops working your baby can be habituated to an interrupted sleeping pattern. It is best to feed in a light sleep cycle for the focal feed. Meaning once you have decided what time your infant will be fed (10 p.m. for newborns – close to midnight or after for 3-4 months of age), you will feed your baby when he naturally wakes in this time range. At this stage, your baby can go approximately 3-5 hours between feedings.
- **4-6 months** – coming up on 6 months you will want the focal feed to be as close to midnight as possible. However, at this time if your baby is already waking consistently at a certain time (say 11:00 p.m. for a hearty feeding), then go ahead and feed your baby. At this stage, your baby can go approximately 5-7 hours between feedings. Many can go 8 hours.
- **6-months** – if by this time your baby has not naturally fallen into a consistent focal feed time that is very close to midnight or after, I recommend that YOU pick a time and stick to it.
- **6-8 months** – If your baby is getting an early morning feeding between 4:00 and 5:00 a.m. this can interrupt night sleep. I recommend removing this feeding by 7 months. To do this you will push this feeding out to a later time each morning until it is after 6:00 a.m. Once this feeding is at 6:00 a.m. or after, you will want to offer this feeding AWAY from the sleep area and more connected with breakfast time.

1. Tell your child when going to sleep for the night; *I'll feed you after X o'clock.*
2. Feed at any time after the time you decide this focal feed

should be. **Do not wake to feed!**

3. Observe the feeding and see how hungry your child appears. When you put your child back in the crib after that feeding, remind with, *I will feed you again after X o'clock.*

Focal Feed Do's:

- Do consult your pediatrician if you have any questions about weight gain and growth issues.
- Do follow your intuition based on your sensitive observation skills.
- Do not wake for focal feed unless your pediatrician recommends that you do so due to lack of proper weight gain.
- Do remember that this focal feed can be a bit tricky to establish. Many infants fall into it and fit into the guidelines listed above.
- Do trust yourself to know if your baby is hungry.
- Do know that your baby will not starve if you reduce the feedings.
- Do keep track of food intake during the day. Most moms notice an increase in hunger during the day when night feedings are reduced.

Bottles and The Focal Feed

Breast vs. bottle, formula vs. breast milk is a highly charged topic. Whatever you choose is best for you and your baby, all I want to say is – don't feel guilty.

Follow the focal feed directions and offer your baby a bottle at the feeding times recommended for each stage of development.

For different reasons your baby may be exclusively bottle-fed or you are supplementing with a bottle. Be it formula or pumped breast milk, working bottles into the night feeding has its advantages and can make the focal feed and night weaning easier.

Advantages of the bottle:
- You know exactly how many ounces your baby is getting in the night.
- Dad can do some of the night feedings.
- You can reduce feedings in the middle of the night by either reducing the ounces in the bottle or you can reduce the ratio of formula to water.
- The bottle can help parents differentiate needs. Babies tend to use the bottle more for food than for comfort. Most babies don't tend to snuggle up to it and extend their sucking for the other reasons that the breast may offer (bonding, reassurance and connection to mommy)

Many mothers use the bottle in the same way as others use breast-feeding. They let their baby suck to sleep on the bottle. If your baby is exclusively bottle-fed, you will want to offer a few ounces at the beginning of the ritual before bedtime and the remaining ounces after the song or story. This can help your baby in not crashing on the bottle. You will remove the bottle before your baby is fully asleep and put him in the crib sleepy but awake.

Chapter 4

Understanding The Cry –
Without Going Insane!

In this chapter, you will learn:

• Crying is a natural part of learning something new and unfamiliar.

• How to cope with the cry

• How to listen and respond to the cry.

Why it matters:

How we cope with the cry and respond to the cry affects our child's ability to self soothe.

4. Understanding the Cry – *Without going insane!*

Crying is where other programs fail. Avoiding or trying to prevent crying is why parents opt into dysfunctional sleep and opt out of solutions. This is where parents need support and guidance. Due to the Internet, crying and the brain chemistry of crying needs some SERIOUS reframing. This natural part of life is wrongly portrayed as something that damages the growing brain. Nothing can be further from the truth. I would like to take sleep learning out of the trauma model. Time apart from your baby in sleep is neither wasted nor traumatic - unless you insist on making it so.

> *The entire point of this chapter is to change your thoughts and feelings about crying. It is essential that you change your actions and reactions to your baby's cry.*

I would estimate that most (90%) of the support I offer is around one thing - the cry. My goal is to reframe some of your existing beliefs around crying. There is a societal myth that suggests that if we let our children struggle (cry) in their efforts to learn a new skill, then we are damaging the bond and secure attachment they have with us. It takes MUCH more than that to damage an already healthy bond. In fact, my bias is that supporting our children in struggle increases the bond if we do it in a consistent, mindful, and compassionate way. Dr. Allan Schore is a leading attachment theorist in the United States right now and quite possibly the world. His affiliation with the RIE philosophy is an important one. Academics dig him. His research backs up our already existing beliefs; that the well-loved and well cared for infant is resilient and capable. His research is the foundation of my "cry reduction" plan. But most regular people would rather hang from the rafters than struggle through his pedantic, scholarly language. For more information on this topic, read my blog post on Regulatory Theory.

Reframe your beliefs about crying:

- We are not leaving them alone to cry.
- We are coming and going and helping them with emotional regulation. Your baby already has several months of data on your coming and going.
- Every time you leave, you return. Every time he sees the back of your head he sees your face again. You will reaffirm his trust in you as you come and go and support him in learning a new way of sleep.
- We are facilitating the cycling that is described further below.
- They are learning separateness.
- Separateness is very different than abandonment.

Here is what will best support our children in learning that there is safety and contentment in being separate. We must provide an accurate mirror. After giving the gift of the secure attachment, the next difficult job of the parent is to accurately mirror to the child their emotional experiences of joy, pleasure, pain, frustration, and discomfort (just to name a few). This is difficult because for several years they cannot tell us what is going on.

We are the regulatory system for the infant and young child. We are assisting them with emotional regulation for quite some time. What will help the most in remaining helpful and assisting them in self-soothing are the following:

How to assist your child in regulating:

- Responding from a place of self-regulation.
- Self-center – center the self.
- Confidence in your child's ability to learn a new skill.
- The idea that all human emotions are meant to be felt. How you mirror feelings back to your child will teach her that feeling is natural and manageable.
- Understanding what cries indicate struggle and can be listened to from outside of sleep area.
- Understanding what cries indicate suffering and need your presence and your attention.
- You can remain present and responsive without fixing the "falling" of "falling asleep."
- You can help your child soothe without rescuing your child out of struggle.
- You will gain more confidence in which cries can result in sleep and which cries clearly need a calming assistance.

Listening to the Cry Exercise

"Listening to the Cry" is the exercise to help you distinguish between struggling and suffering. It is fundamental to understanding what your baby is trying to communicate and it needs to inform how you will respond.

It is crucial that you do the exercises spelled out in Chapter 5 Self Soothing for Parents. **These exercises are intended to use before and throughout the process of "Listening to the Cry." It will increase the effectiveness of cry reduction significantly. Yes, it will be the hardest part of the exercise. Just do it! Commit to doing it poorly at first. Like parenting, it is a practice.**

<u>**Here is what you need to know:**</u>

It takes from 90 seconds to 21 minutes for a disturbance to pass through the emotional system. (Unless you are neurotic, then it can take 40 years.) The reason it is easier to track in infants and toddlers is because they do not have the one thing that drives, propels, and perpetuates emotional states.

- They do not have a story, narrative, or any dialogue around their experience.
- Their feelings are pure and unencumbered by the story we place on emotions.
- They are in the moment and have ZERO story about the future. This is why they are so happy.
- They are pure sensation. Sensations pass.
- However, they have preferences based on past experience. That is what your child is crying for. She is crying for the one way she knows how to fall asleep. And that is you fixing it.

This is what you will need before you start the Listening to the Cry Exercise:

- A clock.
- A comfortable spot outside of the sleep space.
- A strong and unwavering resolve. Shore up your backbone!
- A sense of your intuition and your expertise on YOUR child.

Listening to the Cry Exercise:

1. **Rate your child's cry from 1 to 10** - 1 is complaining and low-level crying. 10 is a full-on screech fest. I call a 10 suffering but young children are perfectly capable of crying at a 10 and they are still not suffering. However, the parent may well be suffering at that point!

2. **21 Minutes = one full cycle of crying** - This does not mean that you will be listening to your child scream his head off for 21 minutes while you white-knuckle it in the other room.

3. **Assess the cry** - You will be assessing the level of crying in 7-minute increments (7, 14, and 21).

4. **Do your self-centering and self-regulating exercise NOW**! - When we listen to the cry from a calmer place, we start to hear it differently.

5. **Listen for cycling** - Cycle crying is the sound of the brain soothing itself. The cry goes up and down on the scale of 1 – 10. There are crescendos and decrescendos, peaks and valleys to the sound of the cry.

6. **Give the cry some time to cycle** -

   - Newborn to 5 months - allow 2-7 minutes of listening.
   - Older infants and toddlers can take the full 14-21 minutes.

   Remember, you can go in if the cry becomes intense and stays in the high numbers. Otherwise, give the cry 7 more minutes.

7. **When to go in** - When the cry cycles up and stays up at a level 9 or 10 for 5-7 minutes, you can go in and offer comfort, soothing, and support to your child. When you do this you are helping the child cycle down so that he can fall asleep.

8. **Soothe without fixing** - When you go in you will try to do the least amount first. Meaning you will try to comfort and soothe with your voice, touch, presence, and love. These are the sleep associations your child gets to keep.

9. **Hell hath no fury** - At around 6-8 months' parents start to feel like their presence makes the crying worse. This is true.

10. **Don't forget to talk to your child** - No matter how young your child is, get in the habit of saying what you see. Say what you

are going to do. Say what will happen next. Say, *I will be back if you need me.* This is where your mantra will come in handy.

11. **It is helpful if your soothing has the following qualities** - You can start to practice this three-step response to all of your child's disturbances - in the day as well. This way it will look familiar in the night and gives your child a consistent response that they can recognize and rely on:

- Acknowledge – Say what you see. "You are crying."
- Empathize – "I know sweetie. This is hard."
- Reassure – "I will help you."

12. **Walk out of the room** - After you say your sleep mantra you will leave the room.
13. **Start the clock over** - When you leave you will start the clock over again.
14. **Rinse and repeat** - Until your child falls asleep.
15. **DO NOT get hung up on the increments of 7 while listening.** Go in based on what you hear coming from your child – no matter how many minutes or seconds have passed on the clock.
16. **DO add a few more minutes on to your listening when you hear cycling in the lower levels of intensity - (1-7) on the scale of 1-**10.

If you were to graph the cry, 35 minutes of crying may look like this.

Cycle crying, although might hit a high number, has peaks and valleys, crescendos and decrescendos.

Red – High level, go in and soothe
Yellow – Mid level, proceed with caution. Give it more time.
Green – Most likely your child will now go to sleep.

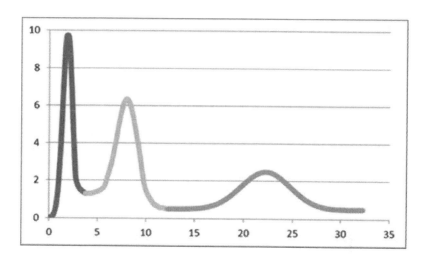

Crying in Real Life

A father's experience: *I thought I was empathizing with her. But I was sinking too far into the pit. I was going to the place of thinking, poor baby this must be horrible for you. It soon became horrible for me too. I realized what she needed most was a strong shoulder to cry on. It was like being in the trenches **with** her rather than being available for her to come up and out. Energetically it felt like a big difference to me. When I made this mental and physical shift I could feel her let go. Soon after I made this shift in my thinking and in my body she went to sleep.*

Email from a mom: *"Eileen, our conversation and your articles have helped ME self-soothe because I understand the crying better. Also, I love that I can go in when he is very upset instead of just based on the clock as typical "sleep training" does. To me, your approach really does feel more connected to the child even though you're showing him he's okay in separateness.*

Though to be honest there hasn't been a whole lot of crying.

I also think doing the story/play prep with Stewie helped me at least as much as it helped him."

As Dan Siegel says, *the story can help integrate the challenging emotional experiences with the other half of the brain so the person can accept the feelings and not panic.*

5 Important Things to Remember About the Cry:

1. **The numbers and intervals of minutes are arbitrary** - Meaning you are going in based on what you hear rather than on the clock. The clock is merely a reality check and a way to see how the crying rapidly reduces in both time and intensity – But only if you remain consistent. The 7-minute cycles are important and you will start to hear the cry decrease if you give it time to do so. The clock will show you "real time" vs. "perceived time." Therefore, the clock offers some objectivity but does not set the hard and fast rule on when to go in.

2. **In the first nights you will go into the bedroom sooner than on later nights.** Once your child learns how to fall (sleepy to asleep in the crib), and where to fall (on the mattress without you fixing it for him), then he understands that he is safe and secure in separateness. Once infants know this we can give them longer to work out their struggle.

3. **The more they do it on their own, the more they <u>can</u> do it on their own.**

4. **As we move forward we go into the bedroom for the big cries, if we feel in our gut they are out of the norm.** We go in more if they are sick or have a fever. We remain responsive and use the above crying guidelines to be less hair-trigger reactive.

5. **We remain an accurate mirror. We do not show up in a panic as if the sky is falling.**

The Cry and Sleep – Two Alternate Approaches

This book outlines my approach to dealing with sleep and crying. In my approach, I am teaching you a measured response, but I would be remiss if I didn't spend some time on the two alternative approaches – neither of which, I recommend.

1. Cry it Out – unnecessary.

If you are reading this book, you probably know about and have already either tried CIO or rejected CIO. My approach offers an alternative. The Compassionate Sleep Solution is NOT a timed approach. You are offering your child comfort and soothing based on what you hear coming from your child NOT the clock. This takes deep listening. Deep listening best happens if YOU are self-soothed and emotionally regulated. I cannot emphasize this enough. You will use the clock mostly as a reality check because 7-minutes sounds like 37-minutes.

2. Stay in the room and "listen till they sleep" approach. *Not* recommended.

Many parents decide that the most compassionate thing to do is to remain in the room and "listen until they sleep." This means they remain a supportive presence for all crying.

Please do not use the method of sitting stone faced in the chair or having your back turned to the child. This will FREAK your child out. Think about it. The cry is supposed to elicit a response. If you are sitting there with a blank face, you look depressed and checked out. This is not good. It is better to be out of the room and come and go.

- If your child has learned that by crying, at some point you give in, because you have in the past, this remaining present and "listening until you sleep" can increase the crying. Who is training who here?
- For this to be successful you will need to work very hard on your own self-regulation.
- This approach works best for newborn to 4 months of age. In fact, this is the only age where I will recommend this approach.
- This approach sometimes works for 4-6 months.
- This approach tends to fall apart any time after about 7-9 months.
- It quits working because your child is too smart. The cognitive awareness at this age is too great. The cry has reached a new level of insistence. Your child knows good and well what the cry elicits in you.
- If you are the object of desire and you are the fixer, then you being present is more stimulating than soothing.
- This is when they tend to cry at us and at an increasingly higher level of intensity. Remember, they have more time and more energy than we do.
- This is when our presence tends to make the crying worse rather than better.
- If you listen until he sleeps then your presence is the new sleep crutch. This can create hyper vigilance in older infants and toddlers. It becomes harder for them to let go and let sleep happen, because when they do, you disappear. This creates constant waking to see if you are still there and calling to you in the night to get your butt in there. *Now!*

- Once the child understands that every time we leave we return, then your child understands that you are reliable and trustworthy. The goal is to create separation *without* anxiety! However, anxiety is a natural part of development and although a parent cannot imagine these two words fitting together – optimal anxiety – this concept spelled out by Allan Schore is what is happening as our children go through the natural and normal increments of anxiety in their development. For more on this topic, read my blog post, Attach This. Your child knows you are coming back because you have NEVER NOT come back.
- This is why coming and going reduces crying.
- Going gives them an opportunity to become distracted by their own sensations and experience.
- Coming back lets them know we hear them and see them.
- This is why coming and going does not damage the bond and cause abandonment, neglect, or trauma.
- Read more about this difficulty in my blog post, Dear Zombie Mom.

The Cry, In Closing

The most important thing you can do around the cry is change yourself. Analyze the cry instead of reacting. This sequence of performing The Listening To The Cry exercise is important:

- Self-regulate. Try not to unravel.
- Respond based on what you hear, not the clock.
- Use the clock for a reality check and to hear progress.
- You will start to be able to make some predictions in the night based on what you hear and the time it takes for your child to cycle down, as in, "I predict that I will not have to drag my ass

in that room because I can tell he is going to go back to sleep in 30 seconds."

When your mind cannot change your heart or your gut, then go to your child. Offer your love and support, just don't fix or rescue. Make sure your tone is one of – *Wow, you are so capable and competent -* rather than – *Wow, you are pleasing me and making ME happy when you go the F to sleep.*

You *can* reiterate to your child how great it feels to give the body this glorious thing called sleep. It is an act of self-love. Therefore, any opportunity we have to turn the child's accomplishments back onto the child the better.

Eventually, the child will come to understand that sleep is something that is done for the self, rather than for the parent. *"You don't sleep through the night because you love me, you do it because you love yourself."* Plus, sleep is one of life's great pleasures. Just ask any cat!

Chapter 5

Self-Soothing For Parents –
Ommmmm...

In this chapter, you will learn:

• How to create the best emotional environment for peaceful sleep.

• Beneficial exercises to help create a peaceful body and mind.

• Your emotional state is a key component of reducing the crying.

Why it matters:

Your child is resonating and tuning to your emotional and physical state of calm – or lack there of.

5. Self-Soothing for Parents – *Ommmmm...*

Your emotional embodied state of how you are relating to your child is the single most important factor of your success in sleep. Who we are and how we show up when we are tired, frustrated, scared and unsure, or confident, relaxed, self-assured and empathetic will be felt by and imprinted into our children. They are tuning forks to our emotional state. They are the most accurate and immediate mirror we will ever place before us. I told that to a dad once and his response was appropriate: "Oh, *CRAP!*"

This is not "woo woo feel good" BS. Mindfulness in this process will reduce your stress about this process. In return, this can and will reduce the amount of crying in your child.

- Mindfulness means paying attention in a particular way.
- When we pay attention in a particular way, we participate in a particular way.
- When we participate in a particular way, we respond in a more effective way.
- When we respond rather than react – transformation is possible.

We tend to do sleep as we have always done sleep. We get tired, we feel sleepiness take us, we fall, and we go to sleep. When we have children we tend to do sleep in whatever way gets us the most sleep.

In the newborn stage this tendency, coupled with the desire to get our baby the sleep he needs, creates the likelihood to fix the newborn/infant's sleep by "putting them all the way to sleep" before we put them to bed.

When it comes to child sleep I encourage parents in practices of mindfulness. This book is designed to walk you through the steps of paying attention to sleep in a particular way.

How you participate in the process of your child's sleep learning will greatly influence the success of sleep in your home. I have learned over the years that the embodied feelings and responses of the parents are what create the prime emotional environment for sleep to happen. OR for sleep to become a disaster.

What are the qualities of mindfulness?

This particular way we pay attention has the qualities of:

- Paying attention on purpose.
- Paying attention in the present moment.
- Paying attention with non-judgment. Judgment in the sense of labeling the experience as good or bad. Good - hold onto. Bad - get the hell away from.
- Regarding thoughts with gentle kindness. Regarding thoughts with gentle kindness fosters an embodied state of equanimity.
- It is a gentle, courageous and purposeful act of awareness.
- We can be aware of our experience and being mindfully aware is a very different awareness.
- We must slow down to become mindfully aware. Fast and quick is how the body does an already learned and well-rehearsed habit.
- Slowing down is a great pace for learning something new. Think snail or tortoise. No one picks up *Flight Of The*

Bumblebee and plays that at full tempo the first time or even the first hundredth time.

- Mindful awareness is a slower pace and may remain a slow pace for quite some time.
- When we think of the baby/toddler perspective, they operate at a much slower pace.
- Observe the pace of your child and meet him/her at this pace and possibly a bit slower in the transition to sleep.

It is a courageous act to become a parent in the first place. It is a very courageous act to allow our children to have their own experience of their struggles in development. For the infant and the young child, struggle most often equals crying. For the parent crying most often equals figure it out and fix it. And fix it equals STOP the damn crying.

Yet we rarely treat ourselves with the same gentleness that we do our children. This equation above sends parents into feelings of guilt and disturbance around the immense amount of emotions the whole process triggers in us.

What gets in our way of this purposeful presence is the narrative that we assign to our every experience? And in my experience there is no louder narrative that takes place than the one that starts to take hold the moment our child starts to cry, complain, scream, and want something from us.

This is full relationship with the self, with the surroundings, with others and with the immediate reality that is in front of us. Bruce Tift in his book *Already Free*, calls this Embodied Immediacy. This is hard. This practice is the hardest when you place something of great importance in that reality. In this regard, that something is our child staring us down and melting our hearts. This practice applied to the relationship of parent/child is both unbearably hard and unbearably joyful. Our children open us up to it all.

Parents often feel self-centered by wanting to have sleep for themselves. They feel that they must put their infant's needs first. Yes, we do put the child's needs first in many regards, but I invite you to look at sleep in this way:

- Giving your child the gift of sleep is putting them first.
- Self-centered is a centered self.
- Centering yourself will help your infant/young child greatly in learning any new skill.
- Therefore, self-centering is a gift to the self AND to our children.

Self-Centering = Self-Soothing

Approaching your child from a centered and self-soothed core will be the best place to offer empathy and reassurance. Anxiety is contagious. We have felt it from being around an anxious person. It is very difficult to hold on to one's center in the presence of anxiety. Infants can feel this as well. Infants are highly attuned to our emotional states, much more than any adult since they cannot counter-balance with thoughts. When we are calm, our chances of calming another are much greater. When trying to calm our infants, being calm is essential.

Self-Centering Practices

Don't just do something; sit there

When it comes to responding to a disturbance in our child, we tend to do the opposite. We do not just sit there, we do something, anything, and if that something has us fixing our child's sleep, we end up down the same old rabbit hole of hopping up every few hours to rinse and repeat.

You must breathe to calm down

Breathe to self-soothe. It is common for a human to stop breathing when agitated or anxious. It is disheartening that the first thing we do when faced with a difficult experience is that we abandon the self. We quite literally hold our breath. This is why I like singing as a soothing activity. If you are singing, you have to breathe. Equanimity is the goal and yet this is incredibly difficult in the face of your crying child. For more read my blog post, Coping with Anxiety Around the Cry!

It seems odd to remind anyone to breathe. However, in this situation I have found three simple breaths to be the most powerful breaths we take in the presence of our children.

This is an exercise I gave parents when I was working on sleep in my RIE classes. I noticed that when parents started talking about their child's sleep difficulties, they would stop breathing. Their bodies tensed and their heads sunk into their necks until their shoulders looked like they were growing out of their ears.

We started practicing this exercise in class and it had a profound effect on the infants. I told parents to go home and do the first part of this exercise for one week. The first part was this and only this:

Just notice what your breath *and* your body does when your child cries.
Don't do anything. Don't try to change it. JUST notice.

- Notice what YOUR body does when your child starts to cry.
- Notice your breath.
- Notice your jaw.

- Notice your facial muscles.
- Notice your shoulders.
- Notice your chest.

Think about holding your child. We hold them at our chest and often close to our face or draped over our shoulders. If we are wracked with tension in this area, they will feel it.

When parents came back to class the following week many noticed that sleep had drastically improved by just changing their own breath and body tension.

Hint: Dads are often better at this than moms. Dads tend to have a different reaction to a baby cry. This is normal. Mom, don't start ragging on dad because he is under-reacting. He is not, but it may look like that in the face of a mother's overreaction.

Here is an exercise that will calm you down so you can provide better support to your baby. This one exercise can change the ease in which your child will go toward a new way of sleep.

Before you go in to support and reassure your child, take two deep breaths and do a quick scan of tension in the areas of your body that I listed above. Don't try to change it and fix it all right there. Just notice - face/ jaw, shoulders/chest, and your breathing.

As you go in to your child, relax into a gentle audible breathing pattern. This is what Dr. Richard Shane calls the "sleep breath." It is the sound of the breathing that you hear when someone is entering into a deep sleep. It is not a Darth Vader helmet breath sound. It is soft and gentle. During the inhalation I think it sounds like a gentle hissing on the back of a relaxed throat and over a relaxed tongue. On the exhale this gentle hiss is heard through the nasal cavity and frontal "mask" of the face.

Remember to look at your child with heavy, half closed and relaxed eyelids, like a contented cat. As our infants imitate facial expressions they also imitate our breathing patterns. Therefore, we want to show them what sleep looks like as well as demonstrate what sleep sounds like. Infants are experiencing all of their senses at once. They are learning everything through sight, sound, touch, and taste. Right now, you are creating a sensual experience using three important senses associated with sleep. Be mindful of what you are putting into your baby in this regard.

If you choose to pick up your crying infant, as you feel his/her body on your own body, breathe into the weight of it. Feel your body melt under the weight of your child's body and breathe into your child. Continue the very soft audible sleep breath and focus on the muscles in your face, shoulders, and chest. With each breath, relax these muscle groups further and deeper. Your intention with each breath is to continually soften the muscles.

Take this exercise one step further, if you wish. If not, that is also fine. The first four steps are enough to create a positive effect.

- Focus on your chest that is now softer and more relaxed. There rests your heart.
- Bring your attention to your heart and rest into that space with gratitude and warmth.
- This experience is an intense and immense heart-opening moment. In this opening we feel deeply vulnerable.
- For many of us it inspires fear and fear leads to other emotions.
- The top two emotions are anger and/or our own tears.
- Be with it.
- It is sometimes painful and sometimes joyful to feel our hearts opening at this depth.

- It is frightening and painful and it is human to want to get the hell away from fear and pain. Remaining present with it is hard. It takes practice.
- It will serve you and your child to begin this practice in your own child's infancy.

I can't remind you to breathe enough. Because breathing is automatic and an unconscious act we become unconscious about it. I am asking you to consciously focus on your breathing when supporting your child in this process. As I mentioned before, one of the reasons why I ask parents to sing instead of talk is because when we are singing we have to breathe. If you are holding your child you can quietly hum your sleep lullaby OR you can just breathe and repeat your sleep mantra a couple of times. I had one dad who simply said...*I know, I know.* I find that phrase to be simple and empathetic.

This empathy we extend to our crying child must be administered to the self. Talk to yourself as you would talk to your child. Be loving and kind to yourself.

We hold this softness - this relaxed and open space for our child. We become the warm and welcoming container for their emotions. We become the anchor of acceptance, empathy, and reassurance.

We show them and share this experience in our bodies.

They can see it, hear it, and feel it. Your child will attune to and resonate with your warmth, empathy, acceptance, and reassurance.

Equanimity: The Mother Of Intention

There are three states of parenting and some would say there are three states of existing in our body/mind/spirit in response to EVERY life experience. We all move in and out of these states. No one state is better than another. Each one is a valid human response. It can be helpful to think of each as an actual physical response to environmental stimulus. Every level of reactiveness, be it emotional, intellectual, or spiritual, can be seen in the following postures:

- Leaning forward
- Centered
- Leaning back

These three states when applied to parenting can become very helpful in sharpening our observation skills. We start to see what our tendencies are and where our habitual responses lie. Below I have added some words attributed to each posture. Although some of the words appear to have negative connotations, they are meant to only describe without judgment or criticism. Each word applied to different situations can have different meanings. Each word could be positive and appropriate in any given moment. Each could be negative or neutral. The point is only awareness. We pause, breathe, and reflect (in RIE it is called the three R's - respect, reflect, and respond). From this place of awareness, we ask the following questions:

- Is this how I want to respond/react in this moment?
- Would a different emotional/physical/mental response serve me better?

It requires a lot of us. To pause when agitated is a very difficult discipline, but it is a worthy practice. It is the grown up form of self-regulation. To keep it simple, these three physical states can be helpful in recognizing when either you or another are in a state of disturbance:

- Leaning forward - Attachment, assistance, interference, interrupting, intervening, facilitating, helping, pursuing, clinging, holding, grasping.
- Leaning back - Aversion, stepping back, moving away from, non-interference, non-intervention, allowing, looking away, tuning out, ignoring.
- Equanimity - Evenness of mind under stress, centered, right disposition, balance, composure, serenity, being with what is, countenance, equilibrium, repose.

My favorite definition of equanimity is this: Emotional or mental stability and composure arising from a deep awareness and acceptance of the present moment.

If our desire is to help our child through a moment of struggle, disturbance, and/or suffering, the embodied state that will serve this purpose most is one of equanimity. The Listening to the Cry exercise is designed to help you in creating this inner state. Any discipline extended from this state of equanimity takes self-discipline. Self-discipline like child-discipline happens with practice and over time. This practice is very, very effective. And at the same time very, very, difficult.

This is important to remember and important to point out.

Equanimity does not necessarily equal a peaceful mind. In fact, it can be quite the opposite. It is remaining present in the face of disturbance. It is remaining present with a non-peaceful mind. And it is NOT a detached approach.

Although I encourage a peaceful body, mind and spirit when achievable, it is expecting far too much of the self to stay there constantly, or even consistently, when we are truly experiencing our child's disturbance. It is acceptance of the present moment. It is hard to accept disturbance, upset, and tears in our child at any moment.

71

Equanimity is abiding in the experience without believing judgments about it. We stay present with wave after wave of intensity and remain present with the sensations with an open heart and open mind.

This practice takes a lifetime, but we can start at any moment! If you start now this practice will become most helpful in adolescence.

Mantras

Mantra can help with equanimity:

I recommend that parents create a mantra for sleep. This is a short and sweet message that you repeat to your child around sleep time.

How is the sleep mantra meant to be used?

This is the practical, logical, and methodical version of mantra. Mantra is a short grouping of words that we repeat over and over around sleep time. This is something that even the young pre-verbal child starts to associate with sleep.

Mantra has these qualities:

- It is short.
- It is simple.
- It is a cue.
- It is to keep us from engaging too much with language.
- Yet it appeals to the child's rapidly growing understanding of words coupled with action.

The historical use of a mantra:

Classically mantra is part of a ritual. It has significance and a meaning. The significance and meaning varies from tradition to tradition. Many a mantra has a representation of peace and love. I like this in sleep. Any time a human attaches a meaning to a word, repeats that word, does so in a ritualistic way, this can have a powerful effect. It is so because we think it so, we say it is so, and we back it with repetitive actions.

The following is my favorite part of a mantra. This too is practical:

This is the sentimental and lovely part of a mantra. It is something we use for decades. It is something that we come to remember represented a sweet, tender and precious time when we closed the day and our children slept cozily in our cave. Ours is, "Sweet dreams and jelly beans, I love you, goodnight." My brother gave that to my children on a visit when they were toddlers and it stuck. We think of him. We all smile.

So make it something that soothes you and makes you feel delight in the prospect of a day when sleep is no big deal and it is peaceful and lovely. It may be hard to believe this from where you sit now but sleep can and will be peaceful and lovely.

Chapter 6

Make Sex A Priority –
Your relationship depends on it!

In this chapter, you will learn:

• What you already know – sex is essential to aliveness.

• Just because you have a baby doesn't mean your sex life is dead. (After having a baby your sex life might have lapsed into a coma.)

Why it matters:

Reviving your sex life is crucial to the intimacy of your marriage/partnership.

6. Make Sex A Priority – *Your relationship depends on it!*

Dear Human,

I am not a therapist, I am not a counselor and I have zero experience on maintaining a healthy intimate relationship for more than a decade. So why am I commenting on sex here? Because I talk to couples every day that are parents of babies and toddlers and are already concerned about their marriages and sex lives.

Feel free to skip this chapter and/or take it with a grain of salt. But we all love sex and figuring out how to have sex that you love, with the one you love, is as worthy a pursuit as getting your child the F to sleep. Because when your child is sleeping could be the best time to get some space to have some sex. Maybe? Someday?

Warmly,
Eileen

Did you come to this chapter first?

I was going to say, "I bet you are the husband." However, I talk to more women than men and there are plenty of women who are complaining about not enough sex. I am guessing it is an equal opportunity desire. Women have the desire for more intimate sex with our partners.

Remember when sleeping together meant something very different than it does today?

Brain drugs: Your very own internal opium den.

The brain is an amazing thing. We can get high on our own brain chemicals. But as all good highs go, we come down off of the high and reality awaits every drugged out brain. No matter what the drug is, we hit the wall and that slide down into reality can be a rude awakening.

Mothers feel this way with newborn babies. And it is because our brain state is the chemical reaction of falling in love. We are high on dopamine, oxytocin, adrenalin, serotonin (albeit lowered levels of the stuff), and endorphins. This is why at first we can do with less sleep and not getting our own needs met. We are all about the love object. And we have the energy we need to keep putting more into our loved one.

This brain state eventually runs its course. Even with our babies.

This is likely why you just read the rest of this book.

Sex activates these dopey chemicals. Sex gets the joy juices flowing again. Sex cements the pair bonding that produced the very baby that is affecting our sleep and/or sex lives.

Most of our babies came about through the wonderful and powerful human experience of sex. Or in some cases, through the wonderful and powerful science of IN VITRO.

And yet nothing wrecks a sex life more than the birth of a child, or two, or more.
Not for everyone but for many of us.

There is a phenomenon in physics called Pair Annihilation. This is where a particle and an antiparticle come together, annihilate one another, and form other particles in the process. This, applied to marriage and children, is a sad phenomenon.

Do you desire reliably great sex?

What causes the death of sex?

- A lack of quality sleep
- Exhaustion
- Interruptions
- Overwhelm
- Stress
- Resentment
- Anger
- Disappointment
- Contempt
- Fear
- Anxiety
- Expectations (built in disappointment and/or resentment)

Just to name a few.

Back in the day, as in the cave days, men hunted and gathered and women tended to the pack. When I grew up it still looked the same with only slight differences. Apparently, the stress of the homemaker was starting to build, since Valium was being dished out like candy to housewives across America.

Those days are gone. Most of my families are dual income households and one or both parents are working full time, or one is working part time. We are trying to have it all by doing it all.

New Stresses on Marriage

This dual income dynamic is a relatively new phenomenon:

1. Both the man and woman (or woman and woman or man and man) are working and earning. Therefore, both in the partnership have work stress.
2. We are both taking care of household responsibilities.
3. We are both involved in childcare.
4. We are both over extended and overly exhausted.

Night comes, and many couples can't get the rest they need because they are up all night facilitating a child, two children, or three children's sleep.

- When we lose sleep we are not at our best and many of us lose our sexual desire.
- When we are sharing our bed or our partner is sleeping in a different room to facilitate child sleep, couples find that sex becomes non-existent.
- When we add the sharing of responsibilities of finance, childcare, running a household, and self-care, we become overwhelmed.
- When we become overwhelmed we become restless, irritable, and discontent.
- When we become irritable and discontent we share that with our partners.

- When we unload that onto our partners in an effort to make them carry some of our "burden" then we start to feel victimized by our circumstance.
- When we start to feel victimized, we start to build a case against the "other" and the other starts to feel villainized.
- Victims are pissed off people. A victim does not feel sexy. A victim does not look or feel like someone that anyone wants to have sex with.
- Non-villain villainized people are pissed off. Villains can be sexy, but mostly only on HBO and Showtime.

Resentment annihilates passion and desire. The solution. Here again, solutions can be simple and not easy. Remember when sex was easy?

- Awareness of the issue is key.
- Acceptance of how the issue was created (and our part in that) is the major key that will unlock the kingdom of great sex, if your solution is to have more sex and feel closer to your partner. Looking at MY part is the hardest part. This is where we will feel most vulnerable with our partners. This is where instead of, *"Oh sweetie it is ok, I still love you, let me give you a backrub do the dishes and serve you a hot toddy in bed."* we might get a *"YES you have been a major bitch and I don't really want to connect with that."*
- Action is the only way to get to the solution. Action will take a fair amount of courage.
- Courage is being afraid and doing it anyway.
- The solution is MORE sex.
- If you are lucky and your relationship hasn't deteriorated to the point of CPR, more sex will lead to better sex.
- Preparation is key.

It will take effort to retain or regain the passion in your marriage. It is easier to retain.
Depending on how far down the sexless tube you are, it may take more effort to regain.

In my practice many families call several years after we have worked together and deliver the sad news to me:
We are separating. Can you help us with transitioning sleep into two households?

The child-focused family most often does not last. At some point we have to take back the night, take back the self, and have a decent sex life if we want to hold on to the relationship.

This chapter is to shed a bit of light on the partnership that brought these children into this world. I will do so in relationship to development, and how the family revolves around the child/children for 2 or more years.

- We are still developing as an individual. We are growing and changing and yet we nail our partners (not in a fun way) to the identification board like a dried-up butterfly specimen that has reached the end of its life cycle. We treat each other as if we are static unchanging beings.

- Our relationships will continue to develop. If they don't, they die. Not a physical death but an emotional death and the death of all desire and passion.

- Our children will survive the struggles of their own development but not all marriages survive the struggle of early family and childhood. Why is this so? Because this is hard and we are mostly unprepared.

- In my travels of divorce, children, and then another divorce, I have had it confirmed, validated, and reaffirmed. It can partially be traced back to and solved in development.

- Our children are the most accurate and immediate mirror we will ever place before us. If we want to see where we are arrested in development, we must pay attention to our reactions to our children.

- If we are arrested in development it will be very difficult to have a mature, intimate relationship with our partners.

- How we moved to and through the stage of autonomy as a young child is a good predictor of how we will move through the stage of autonomy and individuation as an adolescent and young adult.

- How well we achieved autonomy and individuation is a good prediction of how well we will differentiate as an adult.

- We leave home at the level of differentiation our parents achieved. This level will be a good predictor of how we manage intimate relationship when we partner as grown-ups.

This adolescent stage of individuation is where most grown-ups become quite literally "arrested in development." This adolescent stage is very similar to the toddler stage. If we are mindful of that, we will recognize our children (and self) when they hit toddlerhood and adolescence. We will recognize our partners, too, and if we are mature we will keep our mouths shut about that. If you want to kill some more passion and desire, tell someone what a child they are being. That always makes them adore you (I am being an adolescent and going for sarcasm to make my point). THAT is another intimacy killer. So, if your relationship has slipped that far down the tubes and into sarcasm and unkindness, get help - STAT. Unkindness and meanness are very, very difficult to recover from. You can't un-say stuff and you can't un-hear it. So, if it is really mean or critical, try to think before you say it. If it flies out of your mouth because in a heated moment (toddler tantrum) you lacked the self-restraint to contain yourself (toddler behavior) then apologize IMMEDIATELY! Make it sincere (don't be an adolescent about it) and own your part. Nip this in the bud because over time this will erode your relationship.

Our culture confuses intimacy with enmeshment yet we value individualism.

Therefore, we don't know how to remain autonomous and differentiated when we come into intimate relationship with our partners and our children. We tend to become an emotionally fused unit. We merge.

Emotional fusion can also be referred to as overly dependent or co-dependent.

This is normal in the first months and years of the baby focused family. However, tensions start to rise when this natural enmeshment and symbiotic system of early family gets carried into years of the baby's early childhood. Just as a toddler's growing desire for independence is becoming manifest (hence the word, "No!" repeated about a *billion* times), the natural interdependence of early family life must evolve into more stable and separate orbits.

In other words, everyone starts screaming for some space. If we (grown-ups) do not move with the natural development of the child the whole family can get arrested in an uncomfortable stage that does not fit our true needs. We start to behave like the spot we get most stuck in. Most often we start to behave like children and not in-charge adults.

1. Moms and dads get pissed off because they need more support from one another and yet need more space for the self after months/years of being a fused unit. Either or both can start to push each other away like toddlers.

2. Moms become anxious about separating from the child. Mothers have separation anxiety, too. Our emotions become mixed. We cycle cry.

3. Each or both partners can have separation anxiety when they start to separate from one another. We don't know this and imagine the other is "making" us feel unwanted.

4. Dads are trying to do more and have little to no support. How many "daddy and me groups" are there compared to "mommy and me" groups? How is society looking at the "stay at home dad"? This population in the US alone is well over a million. The rest of the population of men are trying to "do it all." YOU are his support system and you may be already wiped out. Yet he is trying to support the family, be the best dad, the best man, the best husband, the best friend, and the best partner. When you go to ask him/her to do one more thing, give consideration to what he/she is already doing.

5. We all need more support, and most of us do not have extended family or close friends nearby to offer the kind of support a tribe/village/extended family/community did.

Space can make the heart grow fonder.

Many of my clients feel this way after they conquer naps. After your toddler has a two – three hour nap you actually look forward to seeing him.

Once fused, most of us then want some distance and space. Not being skilled in differentiation we act like overtired, cranky toddlers. We slap hands away and become indignant, "I'll do it myself!" We want independence. We want breathing room. That is understandable and yet we push others away to get what we want and that becomes damaging.

When we want to be close again it can be hard to draw the pushed away partner back in. Like the toddler, we may feel a desperate need for help, acknowledgement, empathy, reassurance, and closeness. So it becomes a push-me/pull-you type of pairing.

- Come here and go away.
- Help me and leave me alone.
- I am trying to connect with you, can't you see that?
- I am trying to give you what you want, can't you see that?
- I need some time to myself.
- I need to feel more connected to you.

We are trying to do something that has never been done before. Both women and men are trying to "do it all." We have no role models for this set-up. We are winging it.

We are asking a lot - perhaps too much - from our spouses. We want each other to be the best lover, best friend, best parent, best provider, best man, and best woman. And we want this with little to no backup and support from others. We are coupling and parenting in isolation. I consider a couple trying to "do it all" an isolated unit. And in an isolated system, entropy can only increase.

- The solution takes effort.
- It will be personal and unique for each couple.
- Get creative. Find the time. Make the effort.

- We want the security of monogamous long-term relationship yet we want novelty and passion of new romance.
- There is a good chance, high probability in fact, that whatever newness there was in your relationship has already happened.

Lingerie and sex toys will not save us.

What will save us is:
1. Imagination
2. Enthusiasm
3. Scheduled sex
4. Intentional hook ups with your partner/spouse/mate

In other words, you have got to take the time and make the effort to get it up and get it on.

Be prepared – have a game plan – follow through!

The preparation: You will want to create a physical and emotional environment for romance and sex to happen. Guys – this part is up to you! While women appreciate romance, women are not romantic. Men are romantic.

The dress rehearsal: Do a walkthrough in your head. Imagine how your sexcapade will go. The reason why horror movies are so scary (even though we know good and well a head can't spin on its axis) is because our minds can't distinguish between things that are real and things that are vividly imagined.

Vividly imagine having sex with your partner and how you would like this (or him) to go down.

If this doesn't sound romantic to you then it is up to you to make it romantic. If you have forgotten how, then go online and look for the

10 million suggestions on "how to create romance in your relationship." Start small. Choose 5 out of the 10 million. There are books published in both eFormat and on Amazon on "how to rekindle the spark." These sites alone have enough recommendations for free to get the ball rolling.

1. Prepare for this.
2. Prepare yourself.
3. Prepare your space.

The bedroom is for:

1. Sleeping and sex and THAT IS IT! Get rid of the TV, phones, computers, and devices (unless it vibrates).
2. If you can afford it, hit a hotel once every few months.
3. Romance MUST be manufactured at this point and spontaneity, if you are lucky, will show itself on occasion but most likely that mystery ship has sailed. Get over it, get creative, manufacture some mojo about it, and move on.

IF you are resistant to this idea of manufactured or planned nookie, then take a long hard (honest) look at that, because your resistance is about YOU, not your partner.

The person with the lowest sex drive will determine the amount of sex in your relationship. This is just a fact. If that is you, then take responsibility for that. If that is your partner it will do ZERO good to blame him/her. That will likely push him/her further away. But the sad fact is, it is often the guy. Women just have to show up. Guys have to perform. That's why things like Viagra are so popular. Even a non-responsive woman will get in the mood if you take the time to soften her up.

You can either become resentful or blame your lower drive partner for your lack of sex or you can differentiate and grow up about it. Take responsibility and don't take it personally. Become the person you want to be. This is the person your partner was drawn to in the first place. This means that you take him/her off the hook, quit blaming the other person for what you are or are NOT getting, create some space. Get on with your life and what feeds you.

If after all is said and not done, then you might get a divorce. Until then, do the work on yourself and intimacy will be yours either with your current partner or the next one. That is another hard, cold fact. Clean it up now or repeat it with someone else. Because one thing you get to keep in divorce is every bit of the baggage that you came in with.

IF your feelings are hurt then you may have good reason. That exercise in Therapy 101 of reflecting feelings and the idea that someone can't "make you feel" something is one part true and one part BS. Sitting around saying "I feel ___" and "I heard you say you feel ___." is a good start, but if you get stuck there you can spend the lifetime of a relationship thinking this is the end game. When you are in a relationship the other person CAN indeed make us feel very strong feelings. Call it inspire, call it trigger, call it whatever you want. Pushing buttons. Once felt, then WE decide what we are going to do about it. We can make choices on how we go about that. One choice in response to your own hurt feelings, is the same answer that you just learned in this book:

- SELF-SOOTHE
- Self-center
- Self-regulate
- Get over yourself

You will now do for yourself what you taught your child. And you may have to do some cycle crying to get there. Sometimes our partners cannot soothe us. Sometimes they try and can't. Or they have been doing this in overdrive and they are burnt out. It is best to learn how to soothe the self and not rely on another person for that. This is differentiation. On a good day your partner will show up, support you, and be a soothing influence. But your partner will have bad days and not be able to provide that. Be your own good day and soothe yourself.

A large part of what I do in working with parents and crying is to support them in self-soothing techniques. There is NO WAY to soothe a baby if we are anxious and jacked up inside. Anxiety is contagious. This is the same for your partner. Once we are no longer babies it is NO ONE ELSE'S JOB ON THIS PLANET TO SOOTHE US. It is our job to soothe the self. Only from this place can we be of any use to our partner if they are having an off day. So Self-Soothing 101. How do you self-soothe? Here is a list of ways that can lead to unhealthy habits that make things worse. Are you using any of the following to self soothe? Any of these can kill intimacy and end a marriage:

- Drugs
- Alcohol
- Porn
- Sex with someone other than partner
- Spending
- Buying stuff
- Distracting yourself
- Overworking
- Food

Here is a healthier list:

- Talk to yourself in the tone you talked to your child when you were preparing them for the sleep plan.
- Act as if you have compassion for yourself.
- Act as if you have empathy for yourself.
- Acknowledge your disturbances and reassure yourself.
- Hold yourself with loving thoughts words and gestures.
- Think how you would respond to your child if your child were afraid, upset, hurt or angry. Give that response to yourself. When we are in our most autonomous state, we can then offer soothing to our partner. Supporting one another through this is a loving act. If you do not have a partner, phone a friend.
- Breathe
- Exercise
- Meditate
- Drink lots of water
- Eat healthy food
- Stay away from too much sugar
- Sleep

After you do this if you are still upset then it IS time for the (CIO) – Cry It Out approach.

If you were opposed to cry it out for your baby, I suggest you befriend it for yourself. Because either way, staying together or getting a divorce, you will be doing some serious CIO. Yes, I am talking the 'Ugly Oprah Cry' as my girlfriend calls it. There may even be a tantrum involved. You may need to do it alone or with a girlfriend. This might not be the time to take these tears to your partner. However, it is highly likely that eventually you will have to do this alone.

Yes, you will be left alone. You will be completely alone and left to cry in your crib. You will feel abandonment, you will feel neglect, and if you have old wounds around this you will feel traumatized. Remember how I told you infants and toddlers don't have the one thing that propels and perpetuates emotional states? Well, WE do. Your cycle will likely be way more than 21 minutes. You have a story about your emotions AND you have a story (perhaps a case) about how your partner affects your emotions. Perhaps you even have a story about how your partner is responsible for your feelings. This is part of the case you have built. This is dangerous if you do not plan on or desire getting a divorce.

This is exactly what parents fantasize their child is feeling when the child is crying in the crib. Parents think that their child will feel that the parents don't care, that the parent is neglecting them, that it will affect the bond. THEN most couples turn around and do that to each other. This is classic Psych 101 projection and/or transference. We look at the spouse and say, "YOU are not meeting my needs, YOU are making me feel abandoned, YOU are neglecting me, WHAT you are doing is affecting my attachment to you. Because of how I feel I want to get the hell away from you. You are a bad parent to me. I hate you." Back to Toddlerville.

Do:

- Talk to one another in kind tones.
- Acknowledge, empathize, and hold on to the self when the other gets off balance. Reassure one another because you have faith in each other to handle the struggle of your own emotions, your own development and even your own anxiety.
- Have faith in each other that the other is competent and capable.
- Respect one another's autonomy.
- Get some professional help.

Don't:

- Take what your partner does personally.
- Blame the other for their emotional disturbances.
- Blame the other for your own emotional disturbances.
- Criticize your partner.
- Don't overly rely on your partner to "meet your needs."

Most of this is guaranteed to make things worse. Most of this is an attempt to take our feelings out of ourselves. Unfortunately putting those disturbances into our partner leaves us feeling the same. WE feel alone abandoned and neglected. And we wonder why our partner does not want to cozy up to us. It is because we have reverted to a toddler/adolescent state. THAT is not sexy. Parenting is exhausting and it is most exhausting if we feel like we are parenting our partner.
Parenting a grown-up KILLS desire and sex.

Grow up and do it fast if you want your children to grow up. Keep developing. It is the only way to show our children what maturity looks like.

This is about mature intimacy now. IF you think you are ever going to recapture the opium den, doped out, chemical brain state of new love, then you are delusional. You know one another too well. And the old sayings hold up - *Familiarity breeds contempt. And absence just might make the heart grow fonder.*

Once a relationship has deteriorated into contempt it is almost impossible to return from that damage without professional help.

If you would like the best intimacy and sex of your life, THAT is waiting for you. It comes with maturity, effort, creativity, and intention. It comes with admitting who you are, accepting who you are, and holding on to who you are when you get super close to someone else. Most grown-ups suck at this. And it is why a lot of us unravel when our adolescents start to twist off. It triggers our inner adolescent and we get all "GFY" about it.

- Get some space.
- Become attracted to your SELF again – this is first and foremost. This is a MUST! If you feel like crap about yourself then no amount of validation from your partner will make up for that.
- Become attracted to your spouse again – there is no way this can happen until the above is in full swing.
- Connect with your partner, but do it AFTER you have connected with yourself so that you have someone to bring to the connection.
- Don't rely on old sexual patterns and habits to continue to turn you on. Mix it up and experiment with some new sexual styles. Nothing fancy. Or get as fancy as you like. Just don't rely on the old tricks.
- Don't rely on biology and hormones to drive this train.
- Do rely on your curiosity, your creativity, and genuine interest in your partner.
- Have some retro fun. Get playful and rediscover each other.
- Have sex with your eyes open and better yet have an orgasm with your eyes open. It isn't as easy as you may think, but it is mind blowing.
- Talk about all the sex you would like to have a week before you plan your sex date.
- Share some fantasies with your partner in and out of bed.
- Do NOT say, this is my fantasy with George Clooney or Haley Berry. Not that those are wrong or bad but save that sharing for when you are both feeling a little more confident and secure in YOUR relationship. Make your partner the star of your fantasy.

- You can focus on your own physical sensations and yet if you want to increase the intimacy and connection in your sex life, give that up, let it go, and completely focus on your partner's pleasure. THAT is a massive turn on.
- Just have some sex. Any sex. Even OK sex is better than NO sex.
- In time, okay sex can transform into good enough sex.
- Good enough sex can turn into great sex.
- Mind-blowing sex is still ahead of you. I just don't want you to have to wait until the nest is empty to experience that.
- You MUST start somewhere.

The Need for Shared Space

Ideas:

1. Exchange Dinner and a Movie for No Tell Motel - about the same price.
2. Schedule sex.
3. Separate room devoted to sex – farther from the kids room.
4. Take back your bedroom - Get the crib/kid/co-sleeping out of the bedroom.
5. Arrange a play date for them sex date for you.
6. Personal grooming/preparation – cut a path.
7. Do some outside reading in order to get ideas. How about the Kama Sutra? But do some stretching and limbering-up exercises before trying some of those positions.
8. Talk – but save the discussions about the mother-in-law problems for after the sex.
9. Turn off the internal dialog during sex.
10. Hug and kiss longer and more – no more quick pecks, touch more. The average hug is 4 seconds. Try hugging until you are

calm. NOT until your partner is calm until YOU are calm. Here again: Self-regulate.

11. Role-play and create sexy scenarios.
12. Romantic gestures.
13. Surprise your spouse with something fun.
14. **The quick fix**. You fight. You say something mean. Don't let that fester. Apologize ASAP. Receiver – RECEIVE it. Let it go and move on to solutions. Go back to one and two above.

This is all a very simplified version of a very deep and difficult practice. In fact, it is far more advanced than many of us want to achieve. So, get some help, but I warn you, most couples' therapists are not working in this way. Most couples' therapists are working in the old model of "I" statements. Most couples' therapists are training couples in "other validation." "Tell your partner how you feel and get more validation from one another" or find out your partners "language of love" and then do those things to make your partner feel loved. Active listening, mirroring, techniques in becoming more vulnerable, etc. This is fine for many and it may work. In my experience, it is a band aid for the deeper issue.

If we haven't fully done all of this for the self, then we are looking to our partner to soothe us, make us ok. We are asking them to parent us.

Then we wonder why they don't want to touch us.

Recommended viewings, items, and readings:

- Dr. John Gottman and Dr. Julie Gottman of The Gottman Institute
- Esther Perel – *Mating in Captivity*

- David Schnarch - *Passionate Marriage*
- Sex technique eBooks – You must first admit you might suck at something that might need a good sucking...
- Sounds True – Visit soundstrue.com and search for the keyword "relationship"
- Position a day book
- Astro glide
- Coconut Oil – it is edible and non-fattening.
- Pig mask and a cape

Part 2: Action Plan – 3 Steps To Peaceful Rest

You have learned what you need to know. Now, it is time to do what must be done.

Do not skip answering the questions in this workbook section.

Chapter 7

Create Your Best Sleep Environment –
Both Physical and Emotional!

In this chapter, you will learn:

• How to create the best environment for sleep success.

• Why the emotional and physical environment is important to sleep success.

Why it matters:

Your baby's first understanding of the world is the physical context of the environment.

7. Create Your Best Sleep Environment – *Both physical and emotional!*

There are two environments, physical and emotional. These two environments are the keys to your success. The physical environment is the environment of the house leading up to sleep and the environment of the bedroom and the crib or bed where sleep will happen. The emotional environment is how you and your baby feel in your physical body and mind. If we feel panicked, we will create a stressful environment.

Two sleep environments:
1. The physical environment – where your child sleeps.
2. The emotional environment – the emotional state of the parent(s) in relationship to where their child is sleeping.

The easier of the two to keep stable and constant is the physical environment so we will start there.

The Physical Environment

What is the physical environment?

This is where sleep happens. By about 3 - 4 months your baby is sleeping in many different locations (restaurant tables in a car carrier, shopping baskets in Home Depot), hither and yon, here, there, and everywhere. As your baby wakes up to the world, this comes to an end. What will serve him best is:

1. Consistency in where sleep happens for both nap and night sleep.
2. A peaceful and safe place for sleep to happen with ease.

Why is Physical Environment Important?

- Where your baby sleeps is important to the success of sleep.
- Where your baby sleeps is one of the first associations your baby will have with sleep.
- Keeping the where of sleep consistent will help in establishing and maintaining a healthy sleep habit.
- Keeping the where of sleep consistent fosters security and a sense of safety and confidence in your child. Sameness in the environment is very important for the young child.
- Keeping the where of sleep consistent for all of us is an act of self-care and self-love.

How to decide on the where of sleep?

The following is a self-test that you should do with your partner:

1. *Where do you want your child to sleep? How long do you want her to sleep there?*
2. *Do you want to co-sleep? Sleep in close proximity to your infant/toddler/child but not bed share?*
3. *Do you want the whole family to sleep in the same bed, commonly referred to as bed sharing or the family bed?*
4. *Do you want to sleep with your partner, in your bed in your room and have your child sleep in a crib/bed, in a separate room?*
5. *Do you ever want to have sex again? Probably not.*

6. *Do you want to sleep anywhere in the house, or the planet for that matter, **as long as you get some damn sleep**?*

When it comes to the physical environment of sleep you will want to consider the following:

1. **The physical environment is safe.** I will not go into great depth on this topic. Please do your own research. The Internet makes this part easy and it will also scare the crap out of you. Therefore, you will want to take a decent amount of common sense to your reading as well.

2. **The physical environment is peaceful.** I had a dad tell me that he knew a toddler who had learned to fall asleep on the floor, at the foot of his dad's drum set, at around 10:00 p.m., as the dad rehearsed with his band at night. He thought that was a cool thing and adaptable on the child's part. I thought it was sad and borderline abuse. Peaceful sleep needs to happen in a peaceful environment. It does not have to be perfectly quiet, but come on, *drums*?

The Emotional Environment

What is the emotional environment?

In short, the emotional environment is how you feel and how your partner feels about where sleep is happening in your home. The best emotional environment for sleep is one of peace, calm, and confidence. The best emotional environment is one in which both parents want the child to be sleeping wherever the child is sleeping. This is discussed more in the mindful section of this book.

Why is the emotional environment important?

The emotional environment of sleep is one of the key factors in peaceful and restful sleep. **In fact, it could be the most important factor.**

The parent's emotional state sets the emotional environment of the child. We are their regulatory system. Meaning our emotional embodied state will either contribute to our child's emotional regulation or not.

To sleep soundly, solidly, and peacefully, we must have a sense of letting go and falling into relaxation. It helps to have a sense of emotional peace and calm to be able to do that.

Make your own list of the qualities of inner calm and a peaceful emotional environment. Here are a few suggestions to work with:

- Safety
- Comfortable
- Cozy
- Quiet
- Confidence
- Responsiveness
- Connectedness
- Being able to see your baby
- Being able to hear your baby
- Enjoyment
- A sense of spontaneity in knowing what to do
- Connected to your own intuition
- Freedom from excessive fear and worry

- Freedom from self-judgment
- Freedom from partner judgment
- Freedom from conflict

When it comes to the emotional environment, you will want to consider what most often wrecks it.

Because, face it:

- Peaceful nights are what parents (humans) are craving.
- And crying is what parents are avoiding.

Peace and quiet is what we strive for in our physical as well as our emotional environments.

- Parents are hoping to avoid any negative emotions that arise around sleep at both nighttime and nap time.
- Understandably we want to avoid crying because it feels awful and no one can sleep through crying.
- Crying wrecks both the physical and emotional environment of peaceful sleep.

If there was no crying associated with child sleep or changing sleep, the emotional environment would be, "Yay, sleep!" and, "Can't wait to get me some of that!" If this is how you once felt and if you would like to feel that way again, then keep reading.

1. If that is not even close to the current environment of sleep in your home, then keep reading.

2. If this is how you currently feel about sleep, congratulations, you don't need what I have to offer, YET. If it ain't broken don't fix it. However, what works at one stage can run its course and stop working (see chapter on *Falling* and the fix). If your baby is under a year and you feel the imminent end of the current sleep road you are on, then keep reading.

3. If the way in which you are handling sleep suddenly quits working, and you need to change what you are doing, read on.

4. If your baby's crying breaks your heart, triggers your own crying and wrecks your sleep, then welcome to parenthood and read on.

Like the physical environment you will want to have the following two qualities associated with the emotional environment as well:

1. **The emotional environment is safe.** The message we want to send our children is that no matter where they sleep they are safe. We want them to have the sense that they are being seen (watched over), heard and **attended to**. We are powerful in this regard. If we feel safe about it, our children will as well. Yes, it is that simple.

2. **The emotional environment is peaceful.** For this to happen we as the parents need to feel peaceful about where sleep is happening. WE need to project confidence in our children that they can handle learning this developmental skill with our help and support no matter where they are sleeping. If mom can only feel peace and safety if her baby is within arm's reach, then there is your easy answer of where baby will sleep.

Because in my experience there is no amount of convincing the head to change the opinions of the heart.

The physical environment of the "where" of sleep affects the emotional environment of how we (the parents) feel about where sleep is happening. Therefore, both the physical and emotional environments are interrelated and dependent on one another to create the best overall environment for sleep to happen with ease.

How to Create the Best Physical and Emotional Environment of Sleep

How parents feel about the sleep environment and where sleep is happening is vital to getting enough sleep.

In the first months of life I am a supporter of co-sleeping. There is an authentic need for the newborn brain to be in close proximity to a grown up brain. It is also practical given the number of times your baby will need to be fed in the night. However, many families put their baby in their own room from day one. This is not a problem as long as mom is ok with this arrangement. There are two types of co-sleeping arrangements:

1. **Room sharing** – This is where the baby is in his own bassinet, co-sleeper, or crib in the parent's bedroom.
2. **Bed sharing** – Commonly called "family bed." This is where the baby is in the parent's bed.

Therefore, in your preparation of the environment, both physical and emotional, you will want to give consideration to the following when it comes to either of the above co-sleeping arrangements:

#1 - Everyone wants everyone there - Everyone wants everyone to sleep wherever it is that you decide sleep will be.

Many families decide before the baby is born that the family will do family bed and bed share.
Many of us decide that our children will sleep in bassinets and cribs right off. For some of the reasons listed below we end up bringing the baby into bed. I call this unintentional bed sharing. This type of bed sharing sometimes works (rock on!) and sometimes it doesn't (we make another choice).

There can be other reasons that bed sharing suddenly makes sense:

- The baby sleeps better next to us or physically connected to us.
- The baby is hard to soothe.
- We do a night feeding and fall asleep and the baby ends up in bed.

The important thing to remember about bed sharing is this:

- Just because you are bed sharing now doesn't mean you have to forever.
- If it is working, do it as long as it works.
- When and if it quits working, I assure you that there is a solution where all of you can get the sleep you need.

But if you or your spouse do not want your child in bed with you, then this is not a good emotional environment for your child. This happens most often because of the following:

- The parents don't know what else to do.

- The baby started in the bassinet and during a feeding in the night mom fell asleep and baby ends up in the bed.
- The parents have tried to do something else (put baby back in bassinet) and the child reacted with upset and tears.
- The parent is afraid to make a change that might cause the child to react with upset and tears.

Is your partner in agreement with how and where you want sleep to happen? This can be an issue for couples. I have had too many clients whose marriages were affected greatly by disagreements in where and how sleep is being done. I have worked with many divorced couples that reported sleep was a major contributor to the ending of the marriage. I do not recommend any parent relocating their sleep to facilitate their child's sleep. Having dad sleep elsewhere is not the best set up for nurturing intimacy in your relationship. However, many couples do make this choice at some point. If this is your choice you will want to discuss it with your partner and put a time limit on it.

- Having the sleep environment free of conflict between the couple is essential.
- Having the sleep environment free of judgment of the other parent is essential.
- Being on the same page as your partner and feeling their presence, as loving support is essential for a healthy sleep environment.
- It doesn't have to be perfect.
- It doesn't have to be forever.
- It does have to be agreed upon and you can reassess at each developmental stage.

- Sometimes just knowing that this isn't forever is all that you need to know to be able to let go and be with the way it is.
- Circumstances will change and you will have an opportunity to make any changes necessary to improve sleep.

#2 – Everyone is getting the sleep they need – It is important that all members of the family (meaning you, your partner, siblings, cats, dogs, hamsters, lizards, fish) are able to get enough sleep!

Everyone in the family deserves restful and rejuvenating sleep. Allowing this is a form of respect.

Quality sleep can happen sooner than you may believe. Decide how long you can wait for it. Everyone is different. Often within the couple each parent is different. This is understandable. Decide how you want to proceed and support one another in the changes necessary for a higher quality and quantity of sleep.

The Lovey – An Environmental Cue that is also an Emotional Cue

Now is a good time to endear your child to a lovey or transitional object as it is traditionally called. Many parents say, "I have tried but she is not interested." This is most likely because *you* are the lovey (love object, object of desire, etc.). If we remain the lovey, then our child will not be inspired or motivated to use one.
There are three stages of what the lovey is to the child. These coincide with development and the lovey becomes more meaningful as your child grows into a toddler.

1. **Infant** – (When you decide it is safe) 4-6 months. At first it is something to quite literally cling to. This helps the sensation of falling.

2. **Later infancy** – 7-12 months - A physical and environmental cue of our love and warmth in the night.
3. **Toddlerhood** – 1 – 4 years – This is the true meaning of the transitional object. It is a transition in play where the play object is an extension of the child and yet the child knows it is make believe. The lovey becomes a way the child can nurture the self (extension of self) in the night.

I have a client in Boulder, Colorado. He is 4 now. He used his dad's shirt as his lovey and he called it shirt. I saw him one day and asked, "Do you still have shirt?" He said, "Yes, shirt falls me asleep." Well said, well spoken. In learning to fall, our child has lovey to cling to. If they still have us to cling to, lovey will hold no interest. What we are saying to the child is this...
Here cling to this. You can cling to me during the day - at night you have Rocky Raccoon.

How do we endear the child to the lovey at this age?

- WE love on the lovey.
- Bring the lovey into the ritual and infuse it with your love and affection.
- Sing to the lovey, kiss the lovey goodnight, and love that lovey.

Some children take to it, some sort of take to it, some don't at all, and either way, when your child becomes a toddler, don't be surprised if lovey gets hurled at your head or tossed out of the crib.
At that stage you will use the lovey in a simple story or later in a play scenario to bring any point home around sleep. My shirt guy above called his sleep story the puppet show (more on this in *Preparation*).

Respect of the sleep environment in a home:

As I say, my bias is to allow children to do the maximum of what they are developmentally capable of. Since the Compassionate Sleep Solution is based in respect I consider allowing every member of the family to sleep all night long a form of respect. If our sleeping environment is causing us to wake our child, or allowing our child to wake us then this is not respectful. If our sleeping environment is preventing us from physical intimacy, then this is not respectful to our partner or ourselves.

Bed is for two activities - sleep and sex. If you are not getting either, then something needs to change ASAP. I urge you to find a sleep environment and way of sleep where these basic needs are met in both you and your partner and the sleep need is met in your child.

Chapter 8

Create A Routine –
Your baby wants consistency!

In this chapter, you will learn:

• Why the routine of the day is important to the sleep process

• How to create the best routine for your child and your family

Why it matters:

Your child understands the day by the consistent routine we offer.

This understanding leads to the child's sense of security and peace.

8. Create a Routine – *Your baby wants consistency!*

The routine of the day is the first stop on your road to success. Think of each point in the routine of the day as a familiar rest stop with picnic tables in the shade and a beautiful view. Use routine to generate tranquility. Create sameness and ritual as part of your routine. Schedule, as in the specific time on the clock of when each event happens, will take shape over time. I prefer routine over a parent-enforced schedule.

Routine Turns Chaos to Calm

The routine of the day is what happens on any given day, in (and out of) your home. It is the order of events that make up your baby's day and night. What will benefit infants and toddlers most, is to work on a dependable, predictable routine from wake up to bedtime. This alone can solve many sleep issues.

In fact, night sleep starts at wake up time:

- The quality and length of night sleep is influenced by the routine of the day.
- The routine prepares our children for all sleep (both naps and night sleep).
- The routine of naps during the day prepares our children for the best possible night sleep.

Routine includes:

- When – This is schedule. This is the time that each event happens. What time do you initiate critical activities such as mealtime, naptime and bedtime?
- Where - This is the consistent physical and emotional environment in which we care for the child around these needs.
- How - How is the consistent way that we offer our support or offer the child the space to achieve, learn and grow without our interventions or interruptions.
- "How" is a balance of 'on their own' and 'with our help." Sometimes it is completely on their own, sometimes it is with a little help, sometimes we do it for them. The less we do for them, the more they can do on their own. But we will always be close by if they need us.

What are the important qualities of the daily routine?

It is important that a routine is recognizable and repeatable. Children learn through association, experience and the repetition of these associations and experiences. Therefore, you will want to give mindful attention to the following qualities in your daily routine:

- Sameness
- Repetitive
- Dependable
- Predictable

- Peaceful
- At the child's pace when possible. Slowing down to meet the child's pace, when and where we can take this time, is a huge contributor to a peaceful outcome.
- 'Wants Nothing Quality Time' and 'Wants Something Quality Time' (more on this in a bit).

Take a moment of thoughtful care in transitions between events - Transitions are challenging for many of us. This is especially true for infants and small children.

Make room to incorporate the child's pace - The infant's world is a much slower pace than the adult world. Keeping this in mind and avoiding a sense of hurry and busyness can bring a peaceful atmosphere into the home.

Remain mindful of creating a routine with flow and flexibility, rather than a rigid schedule - Parents notice that providing this for their children creates a sense of peace in the parent. Suddenly what seemed overwhelming and stressful has a more effortless ease to it, and life flows. Just try it.

What are the essential elements of the daily routine?

Aside from offering a basic structure and security to the child's daily life, creating a dependable, predictable routine around the following basic needs can solve many of the problems associated with sleep.

- **Food** – Eating at around the same time each day based on authentic need for hunger is important in the daily routine. When at home meals happen in the same spot and in relationship with family rather than walking around being hand fed, left alone in a high chair or in front of TV. We want the child to feel the sensation of hunger and then feel what being sated feels like. This will translate into a child who takes care around hunger and checks into their own feelings of hunger and fullness.

- **Love** – Relationship, attunement, and together time is an important part of the day. This is a high quality time when we are connected to and in attunement with our infants and children.
- **Sleep** – It is important to the success of sleep that naps and bedtime happen at the same time each day/night, in the same place, and in the same way. This consistency in sleep prepares the child for sleep to happen with greater ease.
- **Play** - This is balancing the time we spend together in relationship, and the time your child spends in autonomous play or free play that is not directed, commented on or intervened upon by an adult or caregiver. This is child initiated, child directed and child driven play. Think sandbox.

When we are involved in either the transition between these activities, or in the activity itself, it is best if we are 100% present. This is described in depth below under 'Wants Something Quality Time'. When we tune in to our infants we get a better idea of how slow the infant's world is. For some of us this is most challenging.

Why Is Routine Important?

The events that occur each day, that make up the daily routine, are based on the child's needs:

- When these needs are attended to at the same time and in the same manner each day it gives the child a sense of security.
- Routine shows the child where they are and what is happening.
- When the child knows what is happening next, it gives the child a sense of security and confidence in the parent (caregiver), in their environment, and in the self.

Even young infants quickly learn what will happen next. Their world becomes familiar. Knowing that their needs will be met in a timely, loving and peaceful manner allows them to let go and be fully present to all that surrounds them.

That they are busy learning, and being completely available to this learning, fosters a sense of presence, oneness and joy.

Why is routine essential for healthy sleep habits?

- Routine is the inherent structure of the day.
- Structure is discipline.
- Healthy sleep habits are a discipline.
- Discipline in the early years is adminsitered with a light and loving touch.
- We teach our children the discipline of sleep by being disciplined about our own sleep as well as theirs.

When discipline is inherent in the child's environment, the parent can do less, be more present, experience more enjoyment, less stress and the child can learn more.

We can get out of the way and let the routine do much of our work for us.

Wants Something/Wants Nothing Quality Time

These are both key components of daily routine. For working mothers this time is immensely rewarding.

Wants Something Quality Time – This is the time we spend in direct contact and relationship with our child. This is when the caregiver is doing things to, with, and for the child.

Wants Nothing Quality Time – This includes two different elements.
- One is when we are simply with the child, but not directly interacting with the child. This is high relationship time with the other.
- The other is when the child is safe, but separate. This is high relationship time with the self.

If we do our job right with Wants Something Quality Time, then our children are ready for Wants Nothing Quality Time and this is what gives them the ability to be happily alone in their crib at night! Separateness is a healthy part of any intimate relationship. Separateness happens in tiny increments throughout the second stage of infancy, through toddlerhood, into early childhood and on through adolescence. Many of us work on this concept for the rest of our lives.

Our personal relationship with separateness will show itself when we go through these stages with our children. This will lead to parents having their own varying degrees of separation anxiety. We need to be aware of what is our own separation anxiety vs. the child's.

Wants Something Quality Time

This is when the caregiver and child are involved in an activity that has been set up by the caregiver.

These are the moments in the routine when the caregiver wants something from the child i.e., to get dressed, to eat, to be somewhere, to sleep, or to do anything that we either want to happen, or that needs to happen. These are also moments where the child wants something from the caregiver; i.e. to feed, or to pay attention to the child. From either or both perspectives, something is wanted from the other.

Sometimes the wants of the caregiver are in harmony with the child. These are those wonderful synchronistic moments where we are both involved in an element of the routine and in peaceful harmony, or shared raucous joy.

Sometimes, the wants or need of both (the parent/child or caregiver/child dyad) are not in harmony. For example, the mother knows her baby is tired and needs a nap, and the child seemingly does not agree that this is what needs to happen just yet. The child either wants to continue playing, or has become overtired and is having a hard time letting go and surrendering to sleep. Either way, this can still be quality time, although the latter feels like a lower quality than the more synchronistic and harmonious moments.

In both experiences, the child is learning something of quality and significance. In both experiences, the child is learning about the self, the caregiver, and relationship. In the asynchronistic moments of life, we learn how to deal with the reality of that aspect of life. We learn a lot about ourselves as far as patience, tolerance, and what the lack of a good night's sleep can do to our abilities in that regard. Being aware and present for asynchrony helps us in becoming more appreciative and present in the more synchronistic and harmonious times. Although it is very difficult in the moment, the best action in asynchrony is to become more present in your body and with your child.

Breathe and slow down. This will go a long way in self-regulation and helping your child regulate and settle into the moment.

The Qualities of 'Wants Something Quality Time':

- This is high presence and high engagement time.
- This is a back and forth.
- This is a physical, verbal and/or emotional conversation.
- This is our part in this quality interaction – presence, attunement, resonance and trust (Dan Seigal's acronym or our PART)

This sometimes includes the following in our involvement:

- Sensitive observation
- Listening
- Respecting
- Allowing
- Responding
- Assisting
- Intervening
- Interrupting
- Empathizing
- Comforting
- Reassuring
- Reflecting

Not everyone wants constant togetherness and constant contact. In a respectful relationship there is separateness and this holds true even for babies. Separateness is a healthy part of any intimate relationship.

Please note; as much as the human brain is hardwired and programmed to attach, bond and form meaningful relationship there is also a drive toward separateness. Developmentally separateness looks like this.

- Separate – infant to toddler
- Autonomy – toddler to adolescence
- Individuation – adolescence to early adulthood
- Differentiation – adulthood and for the rest of our lives

Sometimes parents feel guilty that they too want some space. When we build it into the routine of the day the child can know what to expect and what separateness looks and feels like. The child can learn that there is safety, contentment and joy in this time.

The newborn stage of development is appropriately a natural state of symbiosis and enmeshment. In this way, we assure a healthy and strong attachment. However, as infants grow, they are in part growing toward a more and more (minutes to hours) autonomous individual. By the time they are in preschool or kindergarten the time away equals half a day and moves toward a whole day by first grade and so on. Infants, toddlers and children are dependent - NOT helpless.

The healthy attachment and secure bond make for healthy and secure separateness. The crawler or toddler moves away with curiosity and enthusiasm because she knows that there are loving arms, and a lap to return to. Quite often they don't even have to look back as they move away. They know we are there. We have her back. This is trust.

118

Coming and going does not break or destroy trust. In fact, it strengthens it.

The developmental process of the child moving toward separateness happens in the following order.

Enmeshment/symbiosis – fetal stage/inutero – newborn (0-4 months)
Separateness – Newborn – infancy (0-11 months)
Autonomy – Toddler – young child (1 year – approximately 11 years)
Individuation – Adolescent (12 years – approximately 24 years)
Differentiation – Adult (24 years – 90 years)

The above developmental process leads to interdependent relationships with others.
Notice that this is about INTER dependent not independent. There is a difference.

For sleep purposes we want to follow this natural developmental drive toward separateness and autonomy. However, we must start from the natural stage of enmeshment so that our infants are secure enough to move away from us when ready.

Newborn Enmeshment – leads to - secure attachment.
Autonomy - leads to - awesome sleep for the whole family.

Wants Nothing Quality Time

How to do Wants Nothing Quality Time

'Wants nothing time' is when neither the caregiver nor the child wants anything from the other. These times may feel few and far between, but as the child develops this time can be built into the routine to build autonomy.

Wants nothing quality time can be quality time with the self or with the other. Both are important in this process.

With the other, it is simply being with one another and not necessarily doing anything.

With the self, it is when we are physically separate from one another and the child is engaged in open ended, free play, in close proximity, but not in direct relationship or engagement with the parent.

During this 'wants nothing' quality of time, the caregiver is available and present for the child but not directing the activity. From this place of high presence, we can start to build the muscle of autonomy in even our very young infants. Meaning that, the child can have quality time alone. This autonomy quickly turns into autonomous play.

In general, autonomous time alone is best handled AFTER the basic needs have been met.

Here again, sometimes our wanting nothing from the other is a harmonious dance where we go off to separate corners of the dance floor, and groove to our own beat. Other times, not so much. Perhaps the parent wants a shower, or the peace and quiet of a hot bath WITHOUT an audience. Sometimes they are our life's little serenity busters. Therefore, we build this muscle of autonomy and grab the moments when we can. Or not. It is up to you and what you believe your infant is capable of, and when. There is no hurry, and in this regard if we tune into the child he will tell us just how much autonomy he can handle, and when the best times are in the routine to handle it.

Fed, slept, loved – leads to – the ability to cope in autonomy.

The qualities of Wants Nothing Quality Time:

- This is high presence and low engagement time.
- When the caregiver/parent is in the presence of the child we are not multitasking. We are not engaged in an electronic device or busying ourselves with another activity.
- When we want to do something else or need to accomplish another task, this is best done separate from the child.
- We always tell the child when we are leaving their presence, even if they are involved in play or happily looking away.
- Leaving without telling the child or sneaking out creates insecurity and hyper-vigilance in the child. If the child is in a stage of separation anxiety it is always best to be honest about the separation and make it clear when you are returning. Leaving unannounced increases anxiety.
- From a place of high presence we can move into autonomous moments.
- Respectfully and honestly making it clear that we are moving into a separate autonomy from this high presence time helps to build the child's ability to count on togetherness, as well as recognize and relax into separateness.
- This quality of together time, to the movement apart, then back together again, will prepare our infants for us coming and going.
- This coming and going will prepare our infants to trust that every time they see us walk away, they see us return.
- This will prepare your infants for feeling safe in the space of autonomous sleep.

- If your child is an early riser, it is preparation for you to get an extra hour while your baby happily wakes in his crib or sleep space alone.
- It is best if both togetherness and separate time is built into the routine.
- This is mutuality.
- This is interdependence.
- This is a healthy part of any relationship.

Both 'wants something time' and 'wants nothing time' teaches the child in the way children learn best:

- Children learn best in relationship and through an honest exchange.
- Both teach mutuality, interdependency, and respect of the other as well as the self.

The Routine of the Day – Prepares Your Child For Autonomous Sleep

In my expereice as a sleep consultant and in reasearch as well, our best sleep happens when we are sleeping autonomously. This means when we are alone in a bed and not being touched by children, dogs, cats and even partners.

If you have created the routine I have described up to this point, then you are ready for Autonomous Sleep!

What is autonomous sleep?

- This is the ability of the child to sleep separate from us.
- The ability to fall asleep without our assistance.
- The ability to return to sleep without our intervention and assistance.

Where can autonomous sleep happen?

- It can happen in the the child's own space (bed, crib) in another room (nursery).
- It can happen in their own space in the same room as parents.

What will also benefit your infant and toddler in learning autonomous sleep, is an understanding of daytime autonomy. Autonomy is like a muscle that is developed, with our help, slowly, and over time. Here is where we see our children as individuals. Some infants and children take to this idea naturally and show their desire to be put down and separate from us. Others behave more like barnacles on the mother ship and need more time, gentleness, and care in this autonomy development.

When can autonomous sleep happen?
- Some infants can be comfortable with some autonomy soon after birth.
- Many infants can become comfortable with increments of autonomy in the first 4 months of life.
- Most infants can become very comfortable with autonomy from 5 months on.
- All toddlers can handle autonomous sleep because it is part of their authentic developmental drive.

The progression to Autonomous Sleep:

1. At first our infants sleep in us.
2. Then they sleep on us.
3. Then next to us.
4. Then across the room over there.
5. Then in the next room.
6. Then at sleepovers.
7. Then far far away.

When we offer time during the day without our presence, our hovering, our interaction and our mirroring their every utterence and expression, we show the infant there is safety and serenity in free space, and time alone. At first this may be 5 minutes alone as we go to the next room to fetch a clean diaper. Then it might grow to 15 minutes, to 30 minutes, to one hour, and so on. For some, these extended periods of time can take days or weeks. For other children, the autonomy muscle develops over months.

Examples of Routines

This is a good time to start a daily log of activities. Do write it down but there's no need to get uptight about it. There are simple apps you can use to track your child's routine. Some of these have far too much detail and feel a bit over the top.

You will just want to make a note of the following times of the day when your baby is...

- Hungry
- Sleepy
- Wake ups
- Most active

Here is what to know about routine - it changes with development. The timings are not fixed. These are generalizations and although most infants and toddler fall into certain "norms" at each stage, they are individuals.

What to do when your baby is making a developmental shift?

How do you adapt these routines for your baby?

- Keep track of the day and what happens when. The only way to do this is to have a routine of the day when things happen in the same order every day.
- Remember you need more than one data point to call it a trend. If your baby takes an hour to fall asleep one day/night this does not mean that tomorrow you need to push that nap/bedtime later an hour.
- It is best to make any changes to the sleep routine in 15-minute increments. Every 15 minutes of sleep counts for the brain.
- Most families can find 15 minutes in every routine that can be cut short or cut out altogether.

Example of morning routine for an 8 – 9 month old:

- 6:00 - I hear a wakeful baby on the monitor. She is happy in her crib so I roll over and get on top of daddy (in daddy's dreams).

- 6:30 - Wake up. Wake up ritual, changed diaper.
- 6:45 - Nursed baby out in the chair in the den near kitchen.
- 7:00 - Sat on floor with baby and relished in her well-slept adorableness.
- 7:30 - Mom tells baby "I am going to take a shower and I will be right back." Baby was happy to be in her safe place and moved about to explore her safe and cognitively rich, yet simple environment.
- 7:45 - I hear some squawking coming from the safe place so I check in on my way to kitchen to grab a cup of tea and a piece of toast. I tell her I am going into kitchen I will be back.
- 8:10 - I come back into the den and sit and watch baby while I have my tea.
- 8:25 - I notice she is slowing down, not as engaged in exploring and looking off into the distance (soft signs of sleep). I tell her "I am going to pick you up and take you to your room for a nap."
- 8:30 - Sit in rocker sing a song, nurse her, say the sleep mantra, put her in bed, she vocalizes as I walk out of room.
- 8:45 - Asleep!

How much sleep is needed in a 24-hour period for this age? According to 'The Sleep Medicine and Research Center' at St. Luke's Hospital, Chesterfield, Missouri: 14 - 15 hours of sleep in a 24-hour period. This total number includes both night and nap sleep. Remember that wakeful periods for babies (humans) are normal and that all charts are based on time in bed, not necessarily time asleep.

How naps are placed in the 8-9 month old routine of the day:

Nap #1 begins 2 - 2.5 hours after regular morning wake up.

Nap #2 begins 2.5 - 3 hours after the first nap ends.

- My recommendation is to shoot for the highest number in hours of sleep in a 24-hour period and see where your child falls.
- The total hours of naps for the day should be 3 - 4 hours (for the 4 - 6 month old infant.)
- The total hours of naps for the day should be at least 3 hours (for the 6 - 9 month old infant.)
- By 5 months infants are able to get 3 regular naps that add up to 4 hours of day sleep.
- At around 8 months your baby will transition to two naps a day. These two naps should add up to 3 hours of day sleep.

Nap Schedules

During the phase of sleep learning, lengthening naps, or transitioning to fewer naps, I prefer to base your nap times on the time awake between each sleep period RATHER than the clock alone. Therefore, the schedule below is based on the sleep of a baby who has already learned the skill of falling asleep and returning to sleep without parental assistance.

During the sleep learning phase or when there are any disruptions in your baby's night or naps you will want to base nap timings on the following two factors:

1. Quality of previous sleep period - If there were a lot of night wake ups and disturbances, then the first nap will happen sooner.
2. Number of hours of previous sleep period - if the previous nap was shorter (30 - 45 minutes), then the next nap will come sooner.

To reduce the number of night awakenings and early rising:

- Time awake between end of last nap and bedtime should not exceed 3 - 4 hours. This time can be even less, depending on the child and the quality of other naps that day. During the crawling stage of development, it is perfectly normal for your baby to wake from a nap at 4 and be ready to sleep for the night at 6.

Naps for 4 - 6 month old.

Nap #1 - Begins 1 - 1 ½ hours after rising.

Nap #2 - Begins approximately 1 ½ hours to 2 ½ hours after the first nap ends.

Nap #3 - This is the wild card nap and can begin anytime between 3 and 6 pm depending on the previous naps and quality of day sleep on any given day. This can be a cat nap. Many 4 month old babies are still having 4 naps a day and this is why the last one can fall at around 5 pm and be only 30 - 45 minutes.

If any of the above naps were what I call "crap naps" then you can throw in a 4th nap. This can be a stroller nap or "get it anyway you can" nap. I do recommend using a method other than the sleep crutch you are trying to eliminate.

Bedtime is between 5:30 - 7:30 – This is a big stretch. Bedtime depends on:

- What time your child woke.
- The quality and quantity of day sleep.
- If you are in mid transition to fewer naps.
- Your child's mood and demeanor in the afternoon.
- If your child skipped the afternoon nap altogether.

Sample Schedule of a 5 - 6 month old Baby Who Knows How to Sleep

7:00 - Wake-up. This is the time that YOU decide to go to your child. This is when you do the Wake-up ritual. It is a bright "good morning", tell him how the night went, short and sweet, and involve him in opening the curtains or turning on light.

After the wake up ritual you will do the first nursing/bottle of the day out of the nursery/sleep place in, or close to where meals happen.

You will discuss with your pediatrician when to start solids if you don't have a clear plan for this. There is a current trend now to start sooner based on evidence that earlier introduction of solids lowers later food sensitivities.

8:30 - Nap #1 (start time 1-1.5 hours after rising). This nap is 1 - 1.5 hours in length. One hour after wake up, start to look for soft signs of sleep. To begin nap, you will do a shortened ritual of night time and remain positive, encouraging, and reassuring.

9:30 - Nap over. After nap you can nurse, bottle, solids, whatever suits your child's needs.

11:00 - Nap #2 starts. 1.5 - 2 hours long. The time and length of this nap depends on length and quality of nap #1.

12:30 - Nap ends. Nurse, bottle, solids.

3:30 - Nap #3 starts. It is normal for this nap to be shorter than the other naps. It starts to turn into a catnap at around 7 - 8 months. It can be 45 minutes - 1 hour. The timing and occurrence of this nap depends on first two naps of the day. This is classically the hardest nap of the day. Since your baby will be dropping this nap by 8 months, you can do this one out and about, or in a stroller. If this nap is a bust, push up bedtime. If your baby has consolidated 3 - 4 hours of sleep in the first two naps of the day, then she is ready to drop the third nap.

5:00 - Dinner, bath, lead up to ritual.

6:00 - Bedtime ritual starts. This may include another bottle or nursing.

6:30 - 7:00 - In sleep place, ready to sleep.

You will notice as your baby comes into 8 - 9 months that there will be a transition into 2 naps a day. Here are the signs that your baby is ready to transition into 2 naps:

- The first nap gets a little later.
- The first two naps lengthen to 1.5 or 2 hours.
- The first two naps added together equal at least 3 hours of total naptime for the day.
- The third nap gets harder and harder and is mostly a bust.
- Transitions are hard, and during a transition expect regression, disruption and disturbance.
- This transition can take weeks. Be patient and offer a third nap if either of the previous naps were what I call a "crap nap." A crap nap is a nap that was under an hour.
- During any transition, it is always a good idea to push up the bedtime. This is a classic time for very early bedtime. It is not unheard of to put a baby to bed for the night at 5:00 and have them sleep through until 6:30 in the morning.

Napping Chart

Age	# of Naps	Total Daytime Sleep	Length of Each Nap	Awake Time Between Naps	Notes
0-11 Weeks	6-8 Naps	4-6 – hours or more	10/15 minutes - 4 hours	30 minutes- 1 hour	Naps are all over the place. First brain wake up at 3-4 months can change naps dramatically.
3-4 Months	4-5 Naps	3-4 hours	30 minutes - 3 hours	about 1- 1.5 hours	4-month brain wake up can throw naps off – even for great sleepers.
5-6 Months	3-4 Naps	3-4 hours	30/45 minutes - 2 hours	1-2 hours	Naps start to regulate at this time. 2nd brain wake up very disruptive. Time to work on lengthening naps if infant is stuck in 30-minute catnaps.
7-8 Months	2-3 Naps	3 – 4 hours	1-2 hours	1.5-2.5 hours	Perfect storm of sleep disruptions. 3rd brain wake up, gross motor taking off, dropping 3rd nap.
9-12 Months	2 Naps	3-4 hours	1-2 hours	about 3-4 hours	By this point, your baby should be napping pretty predictably. Development will be the biggest disruption to sleep. Final brain wake up, standing, walking. This is a wakeful brain.
13-17 Months	1-2 Naps	2-3 hours	1-3 hours	3-5 hours	Most babies don't make the transition to 1 nap until close to18 months, so hang on to that second nap as long as you can for this stage.
18 Months- 3 Years	1 Nap	1 -3 hours	1.5-2.5 hours	5-6 hours	Be mindful that your nap is after 12 noon. No more than 4-5 hours between wake-up from nap and asleep time at night.

Chapter 9

Begin With A Dress Rehearsal –
Say it, mean it, show it, do it!

In this chapter, you will learn:

• How to show your baby the new way of sleep

• Why it is important to both you and your child's confidence.

• Children are physical. Showing what will happen is more powerful than saying what will happen.

Why it matters:

When infants and toddlers know what to expect they feel more secure and grounded.

This physical process of preparation can significantly reduce crying.

9. Begin with a Dress Rehearsal – *Say it, mean it, show it, do it!*

The dress rehearsal or 'run through' is how you will prepare your child for the new way of sleep. During the day you will explain and show your child that you are doing sleep a new way and you will guide your child through the new process.

Why is the dress rehearsal important?

This is where you will show your child exactly what the new way of sleep will look like. Preparation is the key to success. Preparing ourselves (reading this book) and then preparing the child is a key component of my "Cry Reduction Program." I have found that this process is as important for the parent as it is for the child. When we physicalize this process we feel more confident in what to do when the going gets tough. Meaning when all hell breaks loose in the night (See 9th Circle of Hell chapter), your body will know what to do because you did this part of the preparation. A properly conducted dress rehearsal can dramatically decrease, and in many cases eliminate crying, particularly in toddlers.

Infants learn everything through association!

Even young infants have learned a lot about the environment where sleep happens. Therefore, the environment is rich in visual cues and emotional cues that help infants understand what is happening: Sleep.

Your ritual will give your child valuable cues to what is going to happen and your dress rehearsal will prepare him for understanding the new ritual and the new way of sleep. The visual and emotional context of sleep is something even young infants understand.

0 – 4 months

There is no dress rehearsal for 0 - 4 months old since we are doing an incremental approach. In my practice I offer a Getting Off To the Right Start package for newborn babies.

I do not recommend any form of what is commonly referred to as "sleep training" from 0-4 months of age. This is not the developmental stage to let your baby do any amount of crying. This is the stage to respond, respond and respond some more. There is plenty of time for learning healthy sleep skills. Use this time to get to know your baby and for your baby to get to know you. What you want most is for your baby to know you as reliable, trustworthy and responsive. There are many things we can do to influence the foundation for healthy sleep habits but they are not covered in depth in this book. Read my blog post, <u>What Babies Know About Newborn Sleep</u> for more information.

5 – 10 months

Even though your baby is still very young, I recommend doing a walk-through/dress rehearsal.

You will talk your baby through the new way of sleep. However, it is important to keep it light on words and more focused on actions and "showing."

Important elements of dress rehearsal:

- This is action based. This is a physical "doing" of the ritual. Show more and talk less.
- Although you are primarily showing the new way in the dress rehearsal, this is a good time to get in the habit of telling your child what you are going to do before you do it.
- As discussed in the ritual section, making the ritual rich with sensory cues (look, sound, and feel) will go a long way in showing this age child what time it is, Sleep time.
- Keep it simple and short.

Good time to endear to a lovey or transitional object:

1. The lovey is something to cling to. As your baby is learning the falling of falling asleep, the lovey is what he can cling to in that transition of falling.
2. The lovey is a visual cue and a reminder of your love and warmth. Therefore, to endear your child to the lovey, you must love on the lovey. This is more than simply holding it when you are nursing. Take the item (blanket, cloth with an animal head attached, or stuffed animal) into the ritual at night. When you sing and snuggle you will sing and snuggle with the lovey. When you kiss your child goodnight, you can kiss this item, say goodnight, and hand it to your child.

There is a huge leap of development coming into 9+ months.

Your baby is starting to understand some words. It is never too soon to start talking to your baby in simple language that tells him what is happening before it happens and as it is happening.

Example of dress rehearsal for 5 to 10 months:

It is best to do this at a time that is unrelated to sleep. Therefore, I do not recommend doing it right before a nap, before lunch, or right before bedtime. You will want to choose a time that your child has had all basic needs met. This is the time when the brain, at any age, is most receptive to learning.

It will be important to present the dress rehearsal when your child is:

- Alert
- Well rested
- Well fed
- Ready for interaction with you

Even though your baby is young, you will want to state that you are going to be doing sleep differently. This is a simple statement. "I have been nursing (rocking, bouncing, etc.) you all the way to sleep. Now we are going to do it a new way."

Then do the following:

1. Sit in a chair or rocker and do the last part of the ritual, that may involve nursing, feeding, singing a little song, etc.
2. Say, "*After this happens I will put you in your crib/bed where you will fall asleep.*"
3. Then, place infant in the crib, and remain still and present for a while.
4. Practice breathing and/or notice how just this act can halt your own breathing.
5. Take a deep breath and then move along.
6. Kiss the lovey, say good night to the lovey and hand it to your child.
7. Tell your child that you will be coming and going from the room to check on her and help her learn the new way of sleep.

8. Then talk to your infant as you go to the door slowly and stand at the door.
9. "I will be out here. If you need me I will be coming back to help you learn how to fall asleep and return to sleep in the night."
10. Do this a couple of times.
11. Come back to the bedside and tell your child, "In the morning I will come and get you when it's time to wake up." (After 6:00am)
12. Take your child out of the bed and go about your day.

Things to keep in mind:

- This does not take long. This process is super simple and super short.
- Remember, your child has experience of you walking in and out of his life.
- This is about separateness, NOT abandonment.
- This is about facilitating your child to learn to become self-soothing.
- This is NOT about leaving him to his own (underdeveloped) devices of forced self-soothing.
- If your child is crawling, then your child has experience of crawling away from you. They happily do this because they know they will come back to the secure base.
- Once we start physically moving in and out of each other's lives your child has data that you are reliable and responsible and you will return.
- A child has to be abandoned to feel abandonment. Abandonment anxiety occurs over time. Not in three nights of coming and going to soothe your child into a new and more functional (albeit separate) way of sleep.
- If you are doing drugs, are drunk, deeply depressed, or randomly leaving the house unannounced for days at a time

and your family does not know when you will be back, then you will want to get help. Stop reading and call a mental health professional immediately. This sets up a child for serious abandonment issues. Your issues are beyond the scope of this book.

- Your child's cries from learning this new way are not cries of trauma and neglect. However, it can feel traumatizing to the adult. Your child is crying for the sleep crutch. You will support him in this wanting and longing to have his sleep fixed for him.
- When you no longer fix your child's sleep for him or rescue him out of sleep then your child will learn how to fall and return to sleep on his own.

Examples of Dress Rehearsal for Toddlers

I am breaking the next phase of toddler development into two stages:

1. Beginning toddler 10 – 15 months or later depending on individual development of the child.

2. Accomplished toddler 15 months – 3.5 years depending on individual development of the child.

The major mark of the transition from beginning toddler to accomplished toddler is when:

1. Expressive language begins and your child is expressing herself with words. Words such as:

   - *"Mommy, help me."*
   - *"Out, OUT"*
   - *"Sleep over"*

- *"Get me out of here!"*
- And the ever-popular, *"NO!"*

2. Another major developmental shift that happens at 15+ months is that your toddler is starting the long process of understanding that others (you, your spouse, brothers and sisters, friends and foes) all have different preferences, ideas, tastes, wants and desires than she does. This will become developed over time. Many adults never fully understand this concept called "Theory of Mind." Well-developed Theory of Mind results in becoming a tolerant and compassionate grown up. It allows us to see other perspectives as valid and at the same time different from our own.

Important Points About the Developing Toddler:

- This is the age where you can start to use story and play to prepare a child for the new way of sleep. What starts as a simple story will evolve into a more complex play scenario as your toddler becomes more accomplished.
- This is also the age where you will clearly and simply state the "problem" with the current way sleep is being done. Toddlers are great problem solvers. In fact, they are seeking problems out as a form of learning.
- This is also the age where, if we have been frustrated and irritated because of the way we have been doing sleep, that we make an amends to our child.
- This is more than an apology. *"I am sorry I yelled at you to go the "F" to sleep."* And if you use constant profanity in everyday conversation, then **stop that immediately!** Apart from causing desensitization, it is not exactly what we want to model. Take it from me. I am a part-time sailor. My kids hate that shit.

- This is about amending our behavior, *"I am sorry. I became angry because I need more sleep. I am going to show you a new way where we ALL get to sleep in this house."*

Toddlers dig feeling competent and capable. Let your child have these feelings. The story and play scenario involves them in a meaningful way that allows them to participate in their own solution.

There are two qualities of the toddler that we want to employ in this play scenario process:

1. Curious enthusiasm - The story we create will inspire this aspect of your toddler. We are simply showing them the new way in a manner they can relate to and with objects they relate with in play.
2. Egocentrism – make it all about them. The main character is your child.

   - Choose an object, a stuffy, or a doll that your toddler plays with.
     - Talk to your child about how and why sleep is not working. Show your child with the toy/doll what it looks like now (the problem or what you are doing that you will not be doing anymore).
     - Show your child what will happen. Show the steps that you will take in the new way of sleep.
     - Then give the object to your child to cling to in the night.

Involving the toddler in this way can reduce tears to none at all and sometimes to an enthusiastic participant in their own sleep solution. Don't hype it. Children are authentic and can see right through that BS.

If your child has not taken to a lovey or transitional object as discussed in the previous developmental stage, this story and play scenario will go a long way in endearing them to the items you use.

In toddlerhood, the transitional object takes on the true meaning of that term. Your child is in an important transition of play. The meaning of this object is this:

1. It is an extension of the child. Children at this age relate to their play objects as an extension of the self. It is why in RIE we do not force them to share these items. They are not yet able to understand this concept. To the toddler it feels like giving away a piece of the self. And since they don't have a true understanding of the future (which is why they are so darn happy), they have no clue as to when they will get it back.

2. However, the toddler understands that this is make-believe. The toddler understands the difference between reality and fantasy. Thank goodness or that Superman cape could become dangerous and would come with a warning "Keep away from tall buildings." However, their feelings associated with both reality and fantasies are real. This object that comes to life through play blends the child, the play, the imagination, and the emotions and helps your child process big transitions and events in his life. Remember your child is learning through play. Your child is learning HOW to learn through play.

Sleep is a health and safety issue. PERIOD!

Once our toddlers are upright and walking we want to present sleep as a health and safety issue. They know we are in charge of this and this is what makes them feel healthy and safe to crawl and then walk away from us.

We change what is not working for the well-being of the entire family. We do it because we love them and we love us. They want the best version of us and in my house that is a well-rested version.

WE make it clear to toddlers that we are changing sleep for two reasons:

1. We can no longer do it the current way - The current way is not working and your child knows that already. We owe it to the child to get honest and show them a way that does work. Some clients come to me because they can't and some come to me because they don't want to. Both are valid reasons to change, and in both, the child can feel the underlying emotions that come from us doing stuff we can't or don't want to be doing. Think about it - how does it feel when someone is doing something they don't really want to be doing? We call that – you guessed it, troops – **work!**

2. Because YOU are capable of more – Toddlers love to be competent and capable. Here again, no hype. We are not trying to convince them they are big boys and girls. They are not. We are simply and honestly saying, "We are changing this because you are capable of more." Toddlers are capable of sleeping through the night. Of course, if they do need us (confusion arousal, fear, illness, etc.) we will respond. Do not try to convince your toddler he is a big boy or she is a big girl. If we frame this as a "big girl and big boy" task, they might need to show us just what a baby they still are. Remember a hallmark of toddlerhood is persistence, resistance and insistence.

Example for Beginning Toddler 10 – 15 Months

Important elements of dress rehearsal:

- This is action based. Even though your toddler understands words, it is important to show more and say less.
- Keep this super simple. Think Haiku rather than children's story.
- As discussed in the ritual section, making the ritual rich with sensory cues will go a long way in showing this age child what time it is. Sleep time.
- Make it enjoyable.
- Give some thought about what appeals to your child.
- If your child is already attached to a lovey or a thingy, use that in the story and play.
- Don't try to hype the new way. We are not trying to convince them how fabulous the new way of sleep will be in hopes that they will jump onboard and not miss the old way.
- Be honest and straightforward.
- Remain matter of fact and nonchalant but do have some fun.
- We are simply showing the child in a way they can relate to.
- The first decade of a child's life is solely devoted to play. We are misguided in our thinking that we grow out of play just because we grow up.

Some examples:

1. What is your toddler into? It is best if the item you use in the play scenario can go in the bed with your child when you are done. However, I have had families use trucks, cars, or trains. One child chose rocks. He had a mommy rock, daddy rock, and baby rock. He would put the mom and dad on the dresser in their room and the baby rock on the dresser in his room.

2. Create a play scenario with this item that will show your child the new way of sleep.
3. If strong emotions have been expressed because sleep has been a problem in your home now is the time to say, "I am sorry."
4. Show the problem. Only show the problem once or twice.
5. After that we focus on the positive.
6. By showing and following through with the new way of sleep we are amending our behavior.
7. Once you show the play scenario you will then do a walkthrough of the scene.
8. Some families combine the play and the walkthrough.

This was one of my favorite scenarios from a client. When they sent a picture of the room there was a tree on the wall with an owl in it. In the child's bed there was a stuffed owl.

It was time for the baby owl to sleep in her own nest.
Daddy owl watched over the forest from the tree.
When baby owl needed him he would swoop down and give her a peck and remind her to go to sleep.
Then the daddy owl would return to his own nest with mommy owl and watch over the forest while the baby slept in her nest.

Then the father tucked her into her bed (nest) with her stuffed owl. And he showed her by going to his room and swooping into her room to give her a peck and then returned to his room.

Super simple.

That night the child fell asleep in her own bed and slept through the night without one tear shed.

This was a child who had never slept alone in her life. All 18 months of it.

- I like nests and caves and dens.
- Lions and tigers or bears can be used in this scenario.
- Cars are in their own garages.
- Trains in their own stations.
- Dinosaurs set up on the floor to serve and protect the sleep place.
- Be creative.
- Make it your own.

Example for Accomplished Toddler 16 months to 4 years old

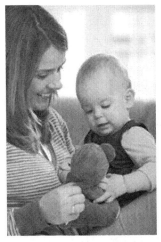

Baby bear woke up and called from his cave in the night. Mommy bear would come in and rock baby bear to sleep.
Mommy bear was so tired she growled..."go to sleep baby bear."
She had to come out of her cave all night long to help baby bear.

It was time for baby bear to sleep in his own cave (make a nest in the crib or bed and show your child where baby bear was going to fall asleep and sleep all night).

This is where baby bear was going to fall asleep and stay asleep all night long.

Mama bear could hear baby bear from her cave

She listened. She gave her baby bear time to lie down and sleep on his own.

Then show the baby bear standing and lying down in the crib.

If baby bear had a hard time, mama bear would come and give baby bear a hug and a kiss.

Then mama bear went back to her cave to sleep.

It is best if this preparation is done under the following conditions:

- A time not associated with sleep – not right before a nap or bedtime.
- When everyone has had all needs met – neither you nor your child is excessively sleepy or hungry.
- There are no distractions and you can be fully present and calm.
- You can use a favored stuffy or doll to show your child the story about sleep.
- Many parents use the template of the story of the three bears similar to the example above.
- Make it simple, short, and all about your child. Your child is the main character.
- This is the time where we start to give the child the problem of the situation if there is a problem. It is OK for your child to know the reasons why you are changing the way sleep is done. Children at any age can handle honesty. Children often handle it better than grown-ups.
- "We can't or don't want to do it this way anymore." is a fine reason.

- You are capable of more. You can do this. We will help you.
- Perhaps there is not a problem with the way sleep has been done until now. If this is the case, then there is no reason to present any problem in the story. Present it with trust and absolute confidence that your child and your family are ready to go to the next phase of autonomous sleep.
- After the story you will do a dress rehearsal of exactly what the new way of sleep will look like in real life.
- If you need to make any changes such as set up a crib, move a mattress, or put up a gate make sure to involve your toddler in this process. Toddlers, even this young, love to be a part of their own sleep solution.
- Let your child see that YOU are enthusiastic and excited about getting more quality sleep. When it comes to self-care we want our children to see us experience the joy of taking care of ourselves.

Chapter 10

Put It All Together -
Opening Night!

In this chapter, you will learn:

• How to create an effective and lasting change in sleep.

• Why your child will come to recognize and soon appreciate the consistency of this approach.

Why it matters:

Life happens and development is ongoing.

Getting off course is part of life.

Getting back to regular and healthful sleep can be a reality by repeating the process you have learned in these pages.

Part 3: Finding Success – Opening Night and Follow Through

10. Put it All Together – *Opening Night!*

If you are going through hell, keep going!
– Winston Churchill

Putting the Pieces Together

This will guide you in putting all the pieces together, creating your plan of action, and moving toward your sleep solutions. It is the ninth circle of hell because no matter what, no matter how much preparation you do, no matter how well you prepared your child, there is no way to know how night one will go.

1. Crying is the hard part.
2. Your fear and story around crying is the hell.
3. You have likely ended up right where you are because you wanted to avoid hell.
4. We all want to avoid hellish experiences. That is human. Get over it and get to the other side of heavenly sleep.

This is what will make hell worse. This is what will keep you in hell.

If you treat each sleep period as a separate and meaningful event, right in the middle of any sleep event, hell can and will happen. It is

149

human to make the prediction that because hell happened at this time in the 24-hour period of sleep, then all other sleep periods that follow this hellish occurrence will be hell as well. If you do this human prediction and projection game - you are screwed. This is when parents stop, return to the old way (sleep crutches) and trade one hell for another hell. As the saying goes, *"Better the devil you know."* **No! This is not true.** Familiar hell is still hell. We think it is better than the unknown hell – that is a lie.

Instead, look at the whole of sleep. See the big picture.

The entire picture of sleep does not hinge on any one occurrence that happens in sleep. And this means sleep heaven as well. If you get high when you are in heaven and low when you are in hell, then you will feel like you are riding a roller coaster and that is its own kind of hell.

It is human to think that improvement will look like this:

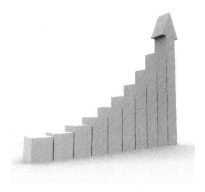

In growth, development and change of habit that kind of continued perfect growth is a fantasy.

Reality looks more like this:

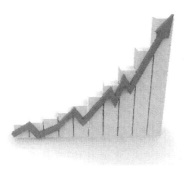

Growth, development, and change of habit are and always will be:

- One step forward.
- Two steps back.
- Four steps forward.
- One step back.

Forgetting is part of the process.

- You will look at the charts above and go...oh, that makes sense.
- You will read.
- You will be prepared.
- You will prepare your child.
- And when the crying starts *you will forget it all*.
- This is normal.
- **This is where you re-read this chapter. Print it out. Post it.**
- **You will sleep again.**

- If you show your child the consistent responsiveness I teach, sleep will regulate and all will be well.
- You will forget that it was ever so bad.
- This too is normal.
- Then a disturbance will interrupt sleep (development, travel, illness, all three at once).
- You will forget sleep was ever good.
- This is normal.
- Forgetting is part of the human condition.
- This is where we re-read and continue doing the plan again and again.

Getting Ready

For this entire process to make sense, you MUST read the whole book. **If you started here first, go back and read this book from the beginning. Everything I talk about below is explained in detail in this book!** Trying to skip that detail is like building a house from the roof down. Please give yourself the foundation first.

Before you begin, take the time to answer the following:

Get out a pen and paper or grab your laptop. Answering the following questions about your process will help you in your actions and the success that follows these actions.

Did you make the necessary changes to your physical environment? Where will your baby sleep?
Do you have a plan for the transition to the next phase of where sleep will happen?

- Family bed to bassinet (still co-sleeping)
- Bassinet to crib in parent's bedroom (still co-sleeping)
- Crib in child's own room
- Bed in child's own room

Are you prepared to create the best emotional environment for Night #1?

- Have you practiced the self-centering techniques?
- Have you practiced this type of responsiveness during the day so that this will look familiar to your child?

Once you begin, it is important to keep on going forward. If not you may end up using the sleep crutches again. This is called...

Intermittent Reinforcement

Dear Parent,

Warning. This next section might make you feel bad. The truth can hurt, as we already know.

I am taking a change of tone here because I really want you to get the concept of intermittent reinforcement.

Intermittent reinforcement and the lack of the parent providing a consistent response for the child, is the one thing that will guarantee more crying when making changes in sleep and eliminating sleep crutches.

Therefore, I want you to sit down, brace yourself, read on and take it like a woman/man. You can handle the struggles of your own realizations here.

I have complete faith in your capabilities.

Warmly,
Eileen

If you walk away from this book with one concept under your belt, let it be this one.

Because intermittent reinforcement is the number one reason for excessive and prolonged crying around changing sleep habits.

Parents call me and a common phrase I hear from mothers is this, "We have tried everything. Sometimes we try everything in one night. None of it works so I end up breast feeding her to sleep and bringing her into bed with me." Often the very baby she is speaking of has been able to fall asleep on her own and then some developmental shift happens and she starts waking more in the night. What is a mother to do?

Quite often parents start to work on sleep and it doesn't go well and by night three they give up. Or it starts off well and a month later something changes and the parent goes back to offering the sleep crutch. Then once they are down the same old rabbit hole it starts to become grim down there. They muscle up and try again only to slip backwards one more time because now the crying is harder and lasts longer. More tears are what they tried to avoid in the first place.

If we offer an intermittent response, then children do not know how long they need to cry in order to get what they want. Remember, crying is easy for them. It is hard on us. They are doing something that comes natural to them - crying. We are fighting what comes natural to us - our drive to fix it and stop the crying.

- Intermittent reinforcement will land you right back in hell. Intermittent reward and response is confusing to the child.
- Intermittent reinforcement is when we intermittently reward certain behaviors in a child.
- In regards to sleep intermittent reinforcement means that sometimes we fix it for the child and sometimes they fall asleep on their own.
- This is the strongest type of reinforcement.
- This reinforcement is the hardest to change.

The behaviors that are reinforced in intermittent reward are the hardest to modify or extinguish. This is because it takes longer to change these behaviors and most often provokes more of the tears we were trying to avoid.

If crying is the way in which your child eventually gets what he/she wants, then at some point you are going to have to break this habit. If we are inconsistent with our approach, then our children do not know what to expect. In other words, if we do not know what we are doing then our children cannot know what to do. If sometimes we fix their sleep and sometimes they do it on their own, this can lead to more wake ups and more crying.

Right about now you may be thinking to yourself, "Does this mean we are going to have to let them "cry it out"? We wanted something different. We do not want to do the "cry it out" method.

Here is why this is STILL not a "cry it out" method or "extinction method." Both which work and there is no evidence either cause any long-term damage or negative effect on the child. I just think this way is better. It is more honest, more positive, allows for two-way communication, it is associated with healthier brain chemistry and the adult remains responsive. This way models healthy relationship. It shows our children that we can be in relationship with them AND their disturbance.

Preparing the child ahead of time is key. We want to be very clear about how sleep will be handled. If there is any apology to be made it is this, "I'm sorry I wasn't consistent and I let you think it was o.k. It isn't o.k. and we are going to change what we are doing." After we show them clearly how the new way of sleep will look, it is the consistency of action that makes the new way of sleep last. Developing a strong attitude that as a sensitive and loving caregiver YOU know what is best for your child will help your inner resolve in carrying out the new way.

Your child has come to expect (and depend on) certain conditions in order to go to sleep. These are often conditions that parents have provided at the expense of their own rest and well-being. On the other hand, perhaps it is not so dramatic. Perhaps you just do not want to do it anymore. Either way your child deserves to know that. You are now modeling healthy relationship by being honest and saying, "We are not willing to continue on this path at the expense of OUR sleep anymore. We are replacing what we did with something new. We will still help you but our help will be different, it will look different, and feel different. Yes, you have an opinion about this. We hear you. We know you want it the old way. Now it is this way."

Here you are modeling to your child how healthy adults with healthy boundaries take good care of the self. The process you are about to enter into is about discipline and boundaries. In the early years, this is done with a very light touch. Yet their response in the intensity of their cry can make it feel heavy and very difficult. With consistency this will pass.

Sleep is a health and safety issue. When you are in charge of this, your child feels healthy and safe.

Intermittency is the biggest reason why parents can't succeed in sleep learning.

Here is why.

Parents perceive that the intermittency is coming from the child. Parents think the child is being inconsistent. This may be true. Given that chart on development in any given moment or "snap shot" of that chart things can look inconsistent, "all over the place" as we put it, or like progress is moving backwards. But this is only if we do not look at those moments in the broader context of change and development. That is only if we are not seeing the big picture.

When we are in the weeds we lose sight of the big picture. And if we are sleep deprived in those weeds we lose touch with reality.

I will tell you now what NOT to do and I rarely tell people what NOT to do. Here it goes.

- Do not look to the child for consistency.

- They are all about change and growth.
- We bring consistency TO the child – they do whatever the hell development is compelling them to do.
- We are the rock – they are the tide.
- We are the anchors – they are the dinghies bouncing around on the waves.

So here is the butt ugly truth of intermittency and what parents hate the most in this truth. **<u>Offering intermittent reward trains the child to cry</u>**. Yes. The loving parent, trying like hell to change something for the better, meets the face of the crying beloved, hands over the boob, sits in the rocker, grabs the baby carrier and fixes the falling of falling asleep. Then when faced with the reality in the light of day we remember – *Oh right that didn't work.* After the horror of that realization the parent redoubles their effort and will try again to NOT do what landed them in hell. The crying becomes louder and lasts longer than it did the previous night. Because by this point the parent has – gulp – deep breath if you are identifying with this nightmare scenario – **inadvertently trained the child to cry.**

I can say it a million times and parents will say, *"Oh right that. Shit. We did it again?"*
- Why?
- What is the block?
- What are we avoiding?
- What uncomfortable truth is this bringing up?

Why? Because we can't handle the crying, we give in and give the crutch. But the crutch quit working. We try one last ditch effort - failed. Hell again. OR we think the child cannot handle the crying. **Why do they block this concept out?** Because it is 2 a.m. and we are exhausted. I mean horribly exhausted, as in close to psychotic exhausted. In this state you become willing to do anything to get back to sleep. That is adaptive and smart on an instinctual level. But it screws your progress up – big time.
What are we avoiding? The F'ing crying that is what. So we give in. And in doing so we create more crying so we give in again. We say we are confused. Maybe but really what we are is afraid. We are afraid to follow through because in this exhausting state we look into this loud crystal ball and see – never-ending crying. And if we have read any of the number of misguided articles on line that do little more than scare

the shit out of parents for allowing a baby to struggle to learn a new skill to sleep, then we are afraid we are doing some irreparable damage. We feel guilty and wrong and like our child will not recover and we give in. Makes PERFECT sense.

What are we really avoiding? We are avoiding sitting tight with our own desire to fix this. We are avoiding our own discomfort over how hard it is to support our child through a loud disturbance. We are forced to sit tight in our own narrative of our own exhausted, disrupted, semi psychosis of sleep deprivation and discomfort and listen to our beloved baby wailing. Oh right and then we are supposed to be "self-soothing". *"She recommends self-regulating and breathing and staying present as this plays out at 2 a.m."* I know. I get it. F me right?

There is no faster way to get a parent to fix something than a story of – *I am a heartless parent I am torturing that child and fucking that child up for life.* That narrative is the good parent's nemesis. And there are plenty of arguments to support that narrative on line. Many of them written by great mothers such as yourself. Great mothers who have needed to find some science to justify their years of sleep disruption martyrdom.

Now wait one second. I have no problem with martyrs. I was raised by generations of good loving martyrs. So let me give you my definition of martyr before I get slammed for being a judgmental bitch.

mar·tyr - märdər/ *noun*
A victim who is proud of it.

And why not. If you are going to disrupt your sleep for years to facilitate your child's sleep, then by all means find some pride in that. And do what I have done. I will bust my own self here because what I have done is human and in some neuroscience circles called a "brain bias".

Find some science to back up your existing belief and way of doing something. And science or pseudo-science is a bone we could pick. But I will not do that here. Maybe in another book.

Much of what I read is not based on actual science. The authors of the red alert, terror wave, of – *cortisol will fry your baby's brain* - try to weave it in but I don't buy it. Because I have woven in my own sciences to back up my own sleep method.

What is presented in blogs and articles, that will scare the shit out of you, on how we must not let a baby cry – ever - in their struggle to learn sleep habits, are (and here is the definition of pseudo-science) a collection of personal beliefs and sleep practices mistakenly regarded as being based on scientific method.

And maybe they are getting great sleep. I believe some people do indeed sleep in a human pile of hot, moving, body parts. I am just here to tell you that for those of us who can't, we are not bad and wrong and messing up our children.

And the family bed is not bad and wrong and messing up their children. But are YOU sleeping? That is the only person who matters in this. Are you and your family members sleeping?
If not.
Then change it.

And yes I am being merciless. I am showing no pity. Because there is a huge difference between pity and compassion. And this is the Compassionate Sleep Solution.

We give over the sleep crutch because we slip into pity. And we are not wrong for doing this.

But pity is different than compassion. Pity is not about the individual who is suffering – the sufferer. Pity is about the person witnessing the suffering. Pity is not being able to contain our own suffering or our own desires to fix the suffering for the loved one. Pity is not having faith in the other's ability to handle this. Pity views the other as a victim.

Empathy is different. Compassion is different. Empathy says, *although I know you can handle this, I will be close and offer you loving support. I will listen. I will remain present and responsive.*

Pity reacts.
- Pity says – Poor baby you can't handle this. I will rescue you.

Empathy responds.
- Empathy says – I hear you baby. This is hard. I will help you through this by remaining calm and present.

Is pity and rescuing wrong or bad? Not always. Just know when you are doing it so you can be conscious about it and choose pity or choose empathy.

Will we have moments of poor baby and dive in and fix it for our little ones? Of course we will.
We are mothers (fathers) goddamn it and we will fix and rescue at some point. And we will have darn good reasons for doing so. And more often we will learn, over time, that when we fix and rescue, it just makes our job harder the next time. And if we do that often then we are creating intermittency and that will confuse our children. Fortunately, time is on our side. These people are not going anywhere for at least 18-years.

I have turned clients away based on their commitment to intermittency. The most recent one was a mom who called me and could not, for the life of her figure our why her 17 month old was still crying at night, all night, and not sleeping. I had to tell her that I could not give her what she wanted. What she wanted was to continue intermittency. This well-meaning, good mother, wanted to nurse her child to sleep at 9:30 (way too late for this age child) and then night wean her for most of the night and then nurse her back to sleep at 5:00 a.m.

I told the mom that this will not work. And here are the reasons.

- The child didn't need food in the night so she was using her breast as the "mommy human pacifier" sleep crutch.
- Therefore, without any authentic need for food the child was just nursing to fix her sleep.
- To tell the child – *OK I will fix it in the beginning of the night and at 5:00 in the morning but the rest of the time you have to fall back asleep on your own* – is unfair.
- In the middle of the night when the child is dazed, sleepy and confused we are telling them "no" when all other times the answer is "yes."

The mother said, "I don't want to confuse her."
I said, "Too late. She is confused. You are confusing her. And this is why she cries every night all night."

This is intermittent reward and the child feels it as intermittent reward and punishment and hence the crying does not stop.

After reading the information about intermittency, it is time to get honest.

Have you tried CIO before and ended up going back to sleep crutches?

If the answer is yes then you may experience more crying.

- Please understand intermittency.
- Don't do it.
- If you are doing it – stop it.
- If you feel guilty as hell right now let that go.
- If you do not think that your child can handle the change and the crying, then by all means don't change. That is fine.
- If you still want to change then let's get on with this show.

This book is the production, I am the producer, YOU are the director, and your child is the actor. The dress rehearsal is an important part of a successful opening night. Taking concepts and ideas and putting them into practice is difficult for any person. I work with hundreds of families who, sadly, have already read several perfectly good books on child sleep. Putting ideas into action and showing the child in a physical way is NOT to be skipped.

Infants:

1. Did your baby watch and participate in the changes to the physical environment?
2. Did you do a walkthrough of the new ritual and show your baby what will be different with the new way of sleep?
3. Are you clear on what times your baby will get fed?

Toddler:

1. Did your toddler participate in the physical changes to the sleep environment?
2. Did you have one last night of doing sleep the old way?
3. Did you make it clear that you are done with the old way?
4. Did you do your play scenario?
5. Do you have your short sleep story for your child prepared as part of the new ritual?

6. Did you do a walkthrough of the new way with your child?
7. Is your child clear that tonight is night one?

First Night

Routine:

1. What time did your child wake?
2. What time did nap #1 happen?
3. Was it a quality nap?
4. Does your child need a second or third nap to make up for any lost sleep?
5. Does bedtime need to be earlier to compensate for any lost or poor quality day sleep?
6. What time will you get home?
7. What time is dinner?
8. What time do you plan on starting the winding down process that leads to the last part of the sleep ritual that happens in your child's bedroom?

Ritual:

1. Do you have a clear picture of your sleep ritual?
2. How long is the ritual?
3. Does it have a beginning, a middle and most importantly – an end?!
4. Is it repeatable?
5. Is it sensually pleasing and relaxing?

Go time!

- The night routine is done.

- The ritual is done.
- Your child goes in the crib/bed.
- You walk out of the door and...
- The crying starts!

What do you do?

Soothe yourself...

Then what?

You keep on going. You come and go. You always have two choices:

1. You go back in and soothe your child.
2. You give your child 7-14 to 21 more minutes and listen for cycling.

What do you do for your child when you go in?

Soothe without fixing it.

Here is what your child is crying for – the sleep crutch.
Your child is experiencing loss and will learn how to replace that loss with something new – his own ability to fall and feel safe in separateness.

Here is what your child gets to keep:

- Your responsiveness.
- Your presence coming and going offering support.
- Your voice.
- Your touch.
- Your face.

- Your love.
- Your warmth.
- Your empathy.
- Your encouragement.
- Your reassurance.
- Your trust in him to be capable and competent at learning a new skill.

All of the above is enough. All children will accept this as enough.

You can do the following to soothe and help your child's cry cycle down. When your child is calm or the crying has reduced you will leave the room.

- **Use your voice first.** Say your sleep mantra. Sing a song. Acknowledge and empathize.
- **Touch your child.** Touch her face. Rub her back. Give her a hug if she is standing at crib side. Hand her the lovey. Rub her head.
- **Sit near and be present** – Only do this if you can remain calm and centered. Pull up a chair and sit close and breathe, sing, or just offer your loving presence.
- **Pick up your child** – If you think holding your child will help then by all means pick him up. You will want to make it clear that when he is calm you will return him back to the bed. As you can imagine or may have already experienced, this can make it worse.

When It's Not Working

The following can happen:

- You go in to help and nothing helps.

- You try to soothe and your child does not stop crying.

Know this, even if your child does not stop crying your presence makes a difference in calming the brain. Just take my word on it.

We come into this world screaming and we kick and scream at varying intensities throughout our entire lives.

When it comes to allowing your child to do something, they are perfectly capable of both developmentally AND emotionally you have two choices:

1. Support them emotionally through their feelings of not wanting change and NOT wanting to do what they are perfectly capable of doing.
   OR
2. Fix it for them.

At different times we will do either of the above. At some point we will do both.
I recommend maximizing #1 and minimizing #2.
If we don't, the consequence is one or both of the following:

1. We lose credibility.
2. We lose sleep.

When your two choices become the double bind:

- You go in and the crying gets worse.
- You leave and the crying gets worse.

This is when you will have to make the choice to go in or give the crying 7-14-21 more minutes. Sometimes going in too often only

stimulates the crying to escalate. The child understands through repetition, "This is working! Gotta do some more."
It is really quite common that the cry goes on for more than one cycle if a child has learned that eventually you will give in and rescue.

How to soothe when nothing works to soothe your child:

If nothing seems to work to soothe your child, then you are going to have to make a decision...

Do I give in and return to the sleep crutch, or do I press forward and trust this will get better each night?

I recommend pushing forward. It will get better.

I recommend continuing to come and go until your child accepts that you come and go in the night just like they accept our coming and going in the daytime.

The most common question about the cry:

This was from a mom who was working on improving the sleep of her 8 month old and 3-Year-old at the same time.

What should we do if they are crying heavily and we are with them, rubbing their backs or talking/singing and our soothing doesn't work? What if they keep crying?
You must breathe and stay present with the cry, walk away from the cry and then return to the cry. If we have fixed a ton of crying by giving into the sleep crutch, then it can send a subtle message that crying is not ok and needs to be fixed. I know it doesn't feel ok.

However, if we know they are not in pain, they are well fed and well cared for and they "want" something rather than "need" something, then remaining with the emotional expression of crying and in a sense becoming OK with their expression is what reduces the crying most of all. We can be doing something that is helpful and being effective and it does not get the results we want in that moment. And in moments of crying, what we want to do is lessen and stop the crying. This will happen. Going through this process and letting the child know that their cries are ok and we can handle them, most often, stops the crying. It takes a few times but it is highly effective.

Chapter 11

Ongoing Success:
Make Naps A Priority –
Never give up!

In this chapter, you will learn:

• Why naps are so important to the growing child

• Why regular and quality naps are harder to achieve than night sleep.

Why it matters:

Naps are important for the developing child for over three years.

11. Make Naps a Priority – *Never give up!*

I recommend that you make changes in night sleep first. Night sleep is easier and the learning happens faster. Once your child can fall asleep and return to sleep at night, she can apply this learning to day sleep.

You will follow the same procedure for naps as for night sleep. But you may feel more discouraged and more impatient about naps. Therefore, I added this section to guide you through naps. Naps feel different and it is because they are different. However, naps still need to happen.

Get to naps sooner rather than later. Stick with it longer than you want. Be as consistent as possible. Naps can happen. It is up to you! Don't let your child decide when nap is over.

Naps introduction:

It is my belief that all children ages 0-3, and some toddlers well into 4 years of age, need naps. For naps to work, even more than in the night, we must become unwavering. Naps are NON-NEGOTIABLE.

Children are learning new skills, each day. This foundational learning of these skills will carry them through life. The developing brain needs regulated and sufficient sleep in order to process, translate, and transfer what is being learned to the area of the brain where memory is stored.

There is a growing body of evidence that children who get quality sleep in the first 3.5 years of life perform better on neurodevelopmental tests at age 6. In these first formative years, sleep will affect your child both cognitively and behaviorally and continue to do so well into the seventh year. This suggests that insufficient sleep during these first few years of life may have long-standing consequences.

Because your child is learning so much in these first four years of life, he needs this time in the day to rejuvenate and rest the brain and body.

There is a wide variety on opinions about naps out and about in your world.

You will meet parents who say, *"Don't knock yourself out. My child doesn't need naps. Yours will be fine."* In this case what most often happened was the child habituated to no naps. What the parent did was follow their child's will out of the crib and out of sleep. We will not judge or criticize. What works for one family may or may not work for another.

I get it. This stuff is hard, but this is a health issue. We do not waver where our child's health is concerned. Don't waver on the nap and the nap will happen. It is true that there are children who are outliers. They need less sleep overall and they do give up their naps earlier than most toddlers. This is not the norm. There does seem to be a link to less sleep and the gifted child. I see this in my practice. The smarty-pants toddler who is speaking in full sentences before two and displaying some pretty advanced creative logic that is fueled by a rise in big feelings and developing emotions can have a harder time turning that sharp and stormy brain off.

The only way to know if your toddler (2.5 and older) is this toddler is to follow this napping protocol and if it does not work after a month or more, then either your child is an outlier or perhaps she has habituated to not enough naps too soon and was unable to shake the habit. Oh well, **make bedtime early enough (asleep by 6p.m.) to make up for this and she will be fine.** Unconditional love overrides EVERYTHING. We will not do this perfectly. Give yourself a hall pass on the naps and hold on to night.

What to remember about naps:

- The first sleep cycle is the shortest. If your child has been waking up after 30 minutes, this was because he could not bridge that first sleep cycle.
- Once a child can bridge this gap then your child can do it more consistently. The next cycle is longer (45-minutes to an hour).

- For toddlers the first sleep cycle can be as long as 45 minutes to one hour and once they go back to sleep they are likely to sleep for another one to two hours.
- In infants and toddler- once naps are stable the combined napping time for the day (1-3 naps) is 2-4 hours total.
- The general rule is the younger the child, the more hours of day sleep they need.
- While working on naps you might need to add an extra nap to get enough day sleep, even if your child has already dropped that extra nap.
- If you must do errands during the first week of this process I want them to be in the morning, short as possible, and preferably after a good nap.
- For toddlers, try to get them home in a reasonable amount of time before nap.
- When children fall fast asleep immediately when the car or stroller starts to move this generally means they are overtired.

- When they wake early from a nap and do not return to sleep

then the next nap will happen 30 minutes – 1 hour later.
- General rule – when naps are crap, push up the bedtime.

The Good, The Bad and The Ugly

Naps: The Good

Once a child learns how to fall asleep and bridge sleep cycles at night he can do it during the day for naps. You are working on lengthening each nap to a minimum 1 hour, preferably to 1.5-2 hours.

Naps happen for a number of years. Once your infant has become accustomed to napping it is easier to hold on to naps during the toddler years.

Good naps make for better nights.

Good naps make for better days.

Good naps make for happier and healthier babies and toddlers.

Naps give you a well-deserved break during the day.

Naps are healthy for the growing brain.

This good news is worth the challenges you have to face to get here!

Naps: The Bad

You are going to want to give up. Don't!

- This is where you will most feel like you are being held hostage to your child's sleep.
- The longer a child has not had a regular napping routine the longer this process will take.
- The more they have been given as far as "facilitation with movement" (stroller, car, swing) or "parental assistance" (crutches), the longer this will take.
- Most often the naps don't regulate because parents give up. Don't quit before the miracle.
- Even the predictable and regulated napping schedule will have hiccups and full on spasms from time to time. Remain calm. Remain on course.
- You have years to work on naps. One bad nap won't spoil the whole bunch but it can make a day feel longer and harder for the whole family.

Naps: The Ugly

Good night sleep is dependent on naps. Naps and night are dependent on one another. If naps don't go well expect a disruptive night. If night sleep was interrupted, make sure ample naps are offered the next day.

If naps aren't working for you and you have tried everything just to facilitate a nap – you need to stop right now! Your child is confused and needs structure.

Why Naps Are Harder Than Night Sleep

Naps take longer to regulate. Here are a few of the reasons why naps are one of the most challenging parts of your child's sleep.

- Naps happen in a different part of the brain
- The drive to sleep is less during the day and the drive to stay awake and be in relationship is greater.
- Your child is learning everything in relationship. Relationship rules the day and she knows well and good that everyone including the dog is probably awake during the day. The older the child, the more they want to stay engaged in play and the harder it becomes to disengage and go to sleep.
- The first signs of separation anxiety can happen right when naps need to become most regulated.
- The older your child is, the more active their brain becomes. It is a beautiful thing and yet your child's brain is lit up like a Christmas tree. In fact, it is a similar brain state as when you were falling in love with your partner. Remember that? When sleeping together meant there wasn't much sleep happening. Your child's brain is like going to Paris for the first time and falling in love on three cups of espresso. When we look that brain in the face and say, "Time for a nap, sweetie," it makes sense that a sippy cup or two will be hurled at your head.

Three Kinds of Naps

Any of these naps can happen EVEN after you have regulated night sleep and your baby/toddler is learning how to fall and re-fall for naps during the day.

1. Good nap – A good nap is over an hour. This means your child successfully bridged at least one sleep cycle and fell back to sleep. If your baby is a newborn, a common practice is to go in and nurse your baby back to sleep after that 30-minute wake

up. This can and does work at first and yet at some point your baby will have to learn to re-fall and go back to sleep on his own.

2. Good enough nap – The good enough nap is about one hour. Sometimes it is not quite one hour but it is good enough to not throw off the entire day of naps.

3. Crap nap – The crap nap is the power-nap that is 20-30 minutes long. They happen in cars often and your baby either wakes up cranky and crying or smiling and flapping her arms as if to say, *"OK good enough. Let's party!!"*

Here is the rule of thumb: If the nap was good to great, rock on. Stay on your routine though. Just because your under-15-month old baby pulled an awesome nap does NOT mean that he does not need that second nap. Stay on your napping routine. If it was good enough, the next nap might happen a little earlier and bedtime still might need to be pushed up based on how well the rest of the naps go that day.

If it was a crap nap, then the next nap will happen earlier AND bedtime will need to be earlier as well.

How to do Naps

Preparation

Preparation is key. Do a new preparation for your naps and follow the preparation portion of this book as described for each developmental stage.

If naps have been handled differently than night sleep you will want to prepare your child for the "new way" around nap.

1. **Say it** - The day before you start your nap plan, in a quiet

moment, tell your child that tomorrow all naps will now be like the night. If you have been using any device to facilitate naps (swing, rock-and-play) then you will want your child to be a part of that item leaving the scene.

2. **Mean it** - The morning you plan on starting on naps, tell your child the same thing in a quiet moment well before the nap.

3. **Show it** – If your child is a toddler this is when you will do the play scenario for how naps will be done. For younger babies a simple story with a lovey or stuffy or just the dress rehearsal is enough to show the new way naps will be done.

4. **Do it** - Then show him/her by doing a walkthrough as recommended in the Dress Rehearsal section of this book.

Nap ritual is a shorter version of the night ritual. If your baby is a toddler you will want to do a nap preparation in story or a play scenario to show her that naps are now going to be like night sleep. Be honest with your child about the problem.

"You are not napping long enough" **Then we show them the solution.** *"The solution is that I'm going to give you more time"*

Your job is to "hold the space" for nap to happen, whether your child sleeps or not. Meaning this - if the nap needs to be at least an hour then at some point your child will need to be in the crib/bed/bedroom for an hour or perhaps more whether she slept or not. We hold the loving boundaries of the following.

1. This is when nap happens.
2. This is where nap happens.
3. This is how nap happens.
4. This is when nap is over and you come out of bed.

Doing this with a matter-of-fact, nonchalant, and laissez-faire attitude will help the most-ESPECIALLY for toddlers.

When nap happens:

Determining the best time to put your child down for a nap is based on three things:

1. Their "sleep cues"
2. The quality of the previous sleep period (night sleep or previous nap)
3. The sample routine
4. The nap chart

Nap Ritual

Short and sweet

This is a shorter version of night ritual. Make closing the blinds or curtains part of the ritual and tell your child, "When the curtains open you can come out of your crib (bed or room)."

After the ritual, sit in the chair next to his crib or bed.

Tell your child, "This is how we are doing it now. You can fall asleep in your crib just like you do at night."

Use your soothing techniques that work at night. When his eyes get heavy tell your child what you see, "Your eyes are closing. I will put you in your crib now to sleep." If your toddler is in a bed you can say, "I can see you are ready to go to sleep now. I love you and will see you after nap."

Put him in the crib/bed and say your mantra or "sleep well, see you after nap." And then walk out of the room.

The Game Plan

Step 1 - Sleepy but awake in the crib and the game plan for naps: Same as night

Use the Listening to the Cry Exercise, and come and go based on what you hear. Since you are working on a shorter period of sleep I recommend going in less. Going in every 5-7 minutes will be more interruptive than helpful.

If you put your child down, he becomes alert and screams, then you say what you see, "You're crying. You are sleepy and you can go to sleep now. Just like you do in the night."

For naps, even more so than for night sleep, I suggest you don't pick your child up unless you REALLY think it will help.

However, if he is still crying at a high level, pick him up and start over again trying to soothe in the crib first and picking him up and holding him in the chair if you must.

If holding was the sleep crutch it will be difficult to use it as a soothing method and having this NOT increase the cry. In this case it is best to do all soothing with the child remaining in the crib.

If soothing and helping your child to return to a lying down position starts to become a wrestling match of up and down and up again, you will say, "My being here is not helping. I'm going to go now and give you a chance to work this out."

Then leave the room.

Give this process 1-1.5 hours.

If you know your child is tired, then he/she does not come out of the crib until nap time is over (1-1.5 hours).

I know this is hardcore. This is hardcore love and although you know this is best for your child, your child will have an alternate opinion.

Step 2 – Come and Go

Since you are working on a shorter period of time I recommend that you come in less often than in the night.

- Remember your baby now recognized this coming and going.
- Remember your baby knows where she is – in the sleep place.
- Remember your baby knows what happens in that sleep place – sleep.

Therefore, this is an environment where she is capable and competent. This is an environment that every day of her life, several times a day, you show up with a face that mirrors the joy to behold her or the concern and empathy of her struggle.

Her data says this – I have NEVER in my life been left here hungry alone in a dirty diaper for hours at a time and no one showed up.

Therefore, I assure you this with the assurance of an arrogant know-it-all.

There is NO WAY your child can feel abandonment, neglect, and trauma because she sees and experiences through the repetitive actions of her day-to-day reality that she has never once been abandoned, neglected, or traumatized. Learning this health skill is not a traumatic process or event.

Do the game plan until it is time for your child to come out of the sleep place.

Do this every day for every nap.

Naps will happen.

Step 3 – Hold 1 Hour Time Boundary

Once we have decided that naps happen, we have to be the benevolent enforcer of the nap. And no matter how loving we are it might just piss them off. See falling in love in Paris above. Remember you know what is best for your child. He needs a rest so he can go another round with his love affair with life and play and the pursuits of development.

1. This is how strong you might have to be. If your child wakes before an hour...wait... listen...rate cry...decide if going in will help.
2. Try to wait 15 - 20 minutes before going in.

3. If you do go in say, "The blinds are closed. It is still time to sleep."
4. Then walk out and wait and listen.

Your child can sleep or make noise but does not come out of crib (or room) until it has been 1 – 1.5 hours.

If nap did not go well and she did not go back to sleep, then take your child out of the crib and you will try again later (15 minutes – 30 minutes)

If your child is a bit wound up from not enough sleep, then it may take 90 minutes for her brain to be prepared to sleep again. Therefore, the next nap may start 1 – 1.5 hours after he comes out of the crib from that crap nap.

Before you take your child out of the room, say, "*It is now after one hour. That was hard. We'll try again later.*"

If your child has shown you that she needs a two-hour nap, then hold the time to 1.5 hours or as long as you can for your child to have the opportunity to re-fall and go back to sleep.

Step 4 – Rinse and Repeat

Please, I implore you, do not base all naps on one bad apple crappy nap.

Desperation can be a gift because it motivates us to change and find solutions in this life. It drives us to a better way. However, it can also lead us to pulling out our bag of worn out tricks and grasping for solutions with the very things that led us to desperation in the first place.

Even after naps regulate a toddler can go on a napping strike. Once verbal they will insist, persist and resist the nap. Out of the blue the upright toddler can rise up and say, "GET ME OUT OF HERE."

Don't freak out.

Hold firm.

Keep at it for a month or more before you decide your child is dropping that nap.

Napping Must Do's:

- **What I recommend and what most parents become unwilling to do - stay home and devote a week or two to naps. This is not forever and yet it is well worth stable naps. I know. It is a drag.**
- Keep activities to a minimum while we are working on naps. Once the naps are regular you will be able to plan the day around the naps. Preferable after a good one.
- **I will repeat** - Since you are working on a shorter time period of sleep, I recommend that you go in less to offer comments and consolations.
- Use only one sleep mantra... *"The curtains are still closed. It is still time to sleep. I'll see you after nap."*
- Your emotional attitude about naps will help immensely or make this extremely tough on all. I get it. This is the hardest part of regulating sleep. I get a bad attitude when things don't

"work out" as I want. Bad attitudes are contagious.

Naps Vs. Night Sleep

What to do about night sleep based on that days naps: Night sleep will become a moving target based on how well naps went. Therefore, expect during the first year that the start of the ritual may need to be earlier when things get funky.

Earlier meaning starting the last bit of the ritual, after bath, in the bedroom, as early as 5:00 – 5:30 so that your baby is asleep by 5:30 or 6:00 for the night.

When naps go well expect a regular ritual start of 6:00 or 7:00 so that your baby is asleep between 6:30 and 7:30 each night.

The goal is to have an asleep time that does not fluctuate by more than 30 minutes on any given night.

Transitioning out of naps

When they don't want to vs. when they don't need to!

Most toddlers go through phases of resisting a nap. Many babies go through phases of simply not taking a nap that they have been taking every day for months. It helps to know this is a normal part of development.

Remember, development alone will disrupt your child's sleep the most. It is important to keep in mind that not everything in sleep is a problem to fix. Some of it will remain a mystery and your job is to continue to show up in a consistent reliable manner.

The ages of nap resistance that are not signs that a child is ready to let go of naps are in early toddlerhood (anytime from 9-months – 2-

years) and then again in later toddlerhood (2 – 3.5 years).

Parents of the 3 to 5-year-old often wonder if their child needs a nap, especially if their child is experiencing significant nap resistance.

How can you tell if your 3 to 5-year-old needs a nap?

I recommend that this determination be made on two things.

1. Your child's behavior,
2. Comparing your child's total sleep time (per 24-hour period) to that of other children the same age.

Signs that your toddler still needs a nap

The signs of insufficient sleep in a toddler can be very subtle and misleading:

- Children at this age who have chronic insufficient sleep may become unusually active, excitable, and appear to be "bouncing off the walls" or wound up.
- Yawning, rubbing eyes, and irritability are obvious signs.
- Being unable to handle a task or situation that your child would normally do with ease.
- Falls asleep in odd places, like highchair or standing up drooped over a couch. Often people send me these Internet pictures as a joke and it breaks my heart to see such exhaustion in a toddler. This level of sleep deprivation followed by literally crashing is unhealthy.
- Immediately falling asleep in the car is another sign that your toddler still needs a nap.
- Accidentally falling asleep in the late afternoon and then having this disrupt bedtime.
- They are hard to wake after an hour and want to sleep 2-3 hours.

- Later in toddlerhood this late long nap can make it very hard for your child to fall asleep for the night at a reasonable time.

The well-rested child appears:

- Alert
- Calm
- Agreeable
- Peaceful
- Content
- Less inclined to tantrums
- Has less accidents
- Engages in less arguments and resistance
- Falls asleep easily at bedtime
- Rarely falls asleep in the car or a stroller

There is mounting research that suggests that sleep loss in the toddler years, even of brief duration, may be harmful for learning. Furthermore, sleep loss is cumulative. Regularly missed naps and going to bed too late on successive days can create a significant sleep debt. In research there is evidence that it not only affects the toddler, but has a negative impact later in childhood.

According to Ronald E. Dahl, MD Sleep and the Developing Brain:
"In specific, cognitive deficits and high hyperactivity scores at age 6 were most strongly associated with a pattern of short sleep duration at age 2.5 years."

In summary, some 3 – 5 year olds need a daily nap while others are able to fulfill their entire sleep requirement at night.

When are we done with naps?

I recommend holding the napping time well into 3 years of age. At first your child may miss one nap a week or more. This does not mean she is ready to transition entirely out of naps. This transition is best if it happens over time. It can take some toddlers 3-6 months to fully transition out of nap. When your child starts to drop the final nap you will want to consider the following:

- Don't call it a nap. You can call it quiet time. You can have specific rules around quiet time such as you must stay in your bed or bedroom and look at books or snuggle your lovey/doll/stuffy.
- If your child falls asleep 50% of the time continue to hold this period of the day for rest and or a nap.
- You will do so for over a month.
- When your toddler starts preschool or any daycare situation she will likely need a nap. It takes a lot of energy for them to hold it together all day for other people. Offer a nap and push up bedtime at the start of any new transition such as school, day care, travel, and major change in your child's life.

If he falls asleep too late in the afternoon, like after 3:00, this is the only time I recommend waking a child from a nap. You will want to open the door to the bedroom and let the ambient noises of the house wake your child after an hour.

This dropping of the nap is where you will seriously need to use your own intuition. Toddlers are ALL very, very different in regards to when nap is over and how that transition plays out over time.

My preference is to let children sleep when they feel tiredness in the body. Don't let them sleep too long or too late if it affects night sleep and don't make predictions for the whole of sleep based on one day or even one week of messed up naps and funky bedtimes.

During this transition as in all transitions it is best to push up bedtime to an earlier point in the evening.

Naps – In Closing

In my work as a sleep consultant, I talk to parents of children of all ages regarding all manner of sleep problems and disorders. I don't think I have ever had a consultation in which there wasn't at least one question on naps.

If I could sum up all of my advice on naps, it would be this – be consistent in the need for naps and in the process of naps even though the frequency and duration of naps change as your child grows and matures.

12. In Conclusion – Nighty night!

During the two decades I have been doing this work, I have had very few families who couldn't achieve the sleep they sought. Most who didn't, wouldn't, and very few couldn't. Those two words are very important to consider.

1. Can't
2. Won't

Often when we say *I cannot*, what we mean is *I will not*.

In most cases the child can and the parent won't. The families who won't 99.9% of the time get stuck on the crying. And they usually end up giving in and handing over a crutch.

We don't hand over the crutch because we are weak (Well, sometimes we are. Sleep deprivation weakens the whole system.) or because we are wrong. We do it because we are exhausted. Your child's brain can handle all of the sleep interruptions much better than yours can. We do it to get the fuck to sleep. (LOVE that book). It is adaptive and intelligent to do the quickest thing to get our grown up brain back to sleep. But doing the quickest thing most often means giving in to the sleep crutch and in the long run we lose more sleep than we gain.

The good news and the bad news is this - it is about the parent and NOT about the child.

There are a handful of babies who continue to cry upon going to sleep for the night and before some sleep periods. Remember, the top reasons for this.

1. Overtired – not enough naps, missing the window of sleep. Or they are temporarily overtired from the process of regulating sleep. Emphasis on "temporarily."
2. Parental anxiety or environmental stress
3. The way some children discharge energy

Other reasons
- Too much travel, especially if it leads to parental anxiety and environmental stress.
- Too many illnesses back to back.
- Too much disruption in the routine.
- Huge developmental leap added to one or more of the reasons above.
- Undiagnosed sensory integration issue.
- Too much intermittent reinforcement. (See above "Before You Begin" section. If you skipped that go back and read and answer questions now!)

Every child is different in their sensitivity to changes and environmental stress.
Children are different in their ability to adapt and handle change.

Common Questions

What if we have a lot of changes to make? For example, what if we are transitioning our baby to his own crib and night weaning and starting a sleep plan? Is this too much? There is never a moment in life that a human is more capable of handling change than in the first 24 years of existence. The brain is changing rapidly and the child is growing rapidly. Therefore, change is a part of everyday life for the child. In later adolescence, change is exciting. Seeking novel experience is part of the drive of the early years right up through the second decade of life.

Therefore, over 90% can get the sleep I promise if they follow this simple and yet not always easy guide.

- You can do this! And when you feel all is lost, you can get it back.
- Crying will happen and yet it won't last.
- Remember you are responding, you are reliable, and your child's struggles will end in the fulfillment of a very important need - SLEEP.
- Your child's struggles will end in a very important life skill – a healthy relationship
- with struggle.

Because of my RIE background, my bias is to allow children to do the maximum of what they are developmentally capable of.

- You are the expert on your child.
- If you do not think, for any reason, that your child can handle the struggle of falling asleep, with your support, but without your fixing it, then by all means wait.
- There is no magic window or stage of development that once passed we will have to nurse them to sleep until they leave for college.
- And yet waiting around hoping your child will "grow out of this" could fall into the category of hopeless hope. Hopeless hope is another word for delusional fantasy.

We can change anything we are doing with our children at any time. ~ Magda Gerber

This takes three things, three ideas, three attitude adjustments, three steps.

1. Awareness – *we no longer want to do it the way we are doing it*
2. Acceptance – *we did it for good reason and now that reason has passed*
3. Action – *we will lovingly and consistently show our child a new way*

Sweet dreams!

Made in the USA
Lexington, KY
19 January 2018